Ultimate Weight Loss

Ultimate Weight Loss Recipes

Table of Contents

Introduction

Low Carb Romaine Lettuce Salad

Chia Seed Dates Oatmeal

Spicy Almond Meal

Spicy Bacon With Egg Scramble

Egg with Pork Sausage Breakfast Skillet

Almond Meal Banana Pancakes

Cinnamon & Pumpkin with Bacon Treat

Easy Lunch Recipes

Low Fat Skinless Chicken Flax Meal

Tuna Sandwich

Low Fat Chicken Cauliflower Slices

Ground Beef Mexican Oregano Fry

Almond Creamy Cakes

Tapioca Nut Spreads

Tapioca Cacao Butter Meal

Lettuce Bacon Sandwich

Ground Meat Long Rolls

Bacon Spinach Salad

Avocado Pickle Relish Sandwich

Broccoli Tamari Nutritional Soup

Sugar Free Raspberry Salad

Low Fat Oregano Caesar

Lettuce Poppy Salad

Green Yummy Pecan Spinach Salad

Veggie Lettuce Gingered Wraps

Celery & Coconut Blend Salad

Crispy Zucchini Rolls

Red Eggplant Pizza

Zucchini Eggplant Dine

Low Carb Chicken & Lettuce Burgers

Spicy Veggie Chicken Breasts Soup

Creamy Coconut Cocoa Fillers

Spicy Ground Beef Medleys

Dinner Ideas

Low Fat Spicy Zucchini

Easy Zucchini Pine Nut Pesto

Zucchini Nut Parmesan Toss

Lettuce Ribs Taco Meat

Orange Creamy Blend

Spinach Shallot Salad

Tomato Dill

Rich Mushroom Stuff

Low Fat Lettuce Gyro Meat Sandwich

Cheesy Macadamia Flax Meal

Spicy Zucchini Almond Crack

Tomato Spinach Pesto

Banana with Pumpkin Soup

Kale Shallot Dish

Low Fat Chickplant Bites

Spicy Roasted Pepper Chicken

Low Carb Basil Eggplant

Orange Zucchini Spaghetti

Fantasy Romaine Lettuce Salad

Coconut Flour Pumpkin Roast

Spicy Cocoa Bread

Low Carb Triple Flour Egg Puddings

Coconut & Almond Teasers

Yummy Chia Seed Flatbread

Quick Asian Naan

All-Natural Baking Recipes

Weight Loss Chocó Vanilla Toss

Low Fat Nut Muffins

Jalapeno Coconut Pretzels

Low Fat Baked Bar with Creamy Topping

Spicy Pepper Biscuits

Spinach Muffins

Sugar Free Almond Slice

Low Fat Tapioca Fillers

Baked Crust Cubes

Yolk Muffins

Low Fat Flax Meal

Gingery Flax Meal

Sugar Free Cream Bread

Low Fat Blueberry Spatula

Chocó Muffins

Almond Pecan Chocó Cookies

Frozen Blueberry Coconut Scones

Low Carb Cinnamon Bites

Almond Flour Chia Bagels

Avocado Bacon Egged Muffin

Coconut Flour Vanilla Muffins

Stuffed Blackberry Almonds

Low Carb Vanilla Dates Bread

Zucchini Egged Cake

Spicy Cocoa Creamy Muffins

Comfort Food Recipes

Low Fat Zucchini Pasta

Creamy Tomatoes

Low Fat Basil Noodles

Nut Nori Dish

Sugar Free Cabbage Bowl

No Cook Fruit Milk

Celery with Cashew Butter

Sugar Free Berry Bars

Vanilla Whisk

Low Fat Nuts Fudge

Dried Apricot Cookies

Cauliflower Saffron Chops

Baked Ramekins

Sprig Muffins

Sugar Free Creamy Chia Cakes

Almond with Apple Sauce – A Low Carb Morning Dish

No Grain Low Carb Almond bread

Low Carb Almond Corn Muffins

Quick Delicious Almond Biscuits – Evening Snack

Coconut & Almond Flour Fry Bread

Crunchy Coconut Crackers

Chocó Dip with Celery

Chocó Pecan Snack

Vanilla Chocó Chip Cookies

Sugar-Free Coconut Ice Cream

On the Go Recipes

Low Fat Apricot Pine Bars

Sugar Free Gingerly Almond Crackers

Dates Almond Wafers

Very Berry Biscuits

Dried Apricot Packers

Sugar Free Creamy Dates Energy Bars

Rich Fruit & Flax Slice

Low Fat Cashew Balls

Whole Flax Orange Crackers

Kale Almond Bites

Triple Berry Flax Bars

Fruit Strips

Carrot Toss Crisp

Mango Mouth Bites

Pineapple Slices

Sugar – Free Crunchy Banana

Low Carb Apple Chips

Cauliflower Popcorns

Spicy Chicken Tubes

Butter Pancakes

Flour Free Egg Toasts

Spicy Pesto Turkey Wrap

Spicy Seafood Wraps

Spicy Celery & Chicken Wraps

Green Spicy Chicken Salad

Quick Snacks

Raw Nut Snack

Creamy Cinnamon Snacks

Apples with Lemon Juice

Energy Reviving Cookies

Strawberry Logs

Weight Loss Tangerine Sticks

Creamy Spicy Onion Bites

Spicy Cauliflower Chips

Weight Loss Flax Crackers

Weight Zucchini Salsa

Quick Weight Loss Dates Spread

All Chopped Creamy Dish

Weight Loss Sweet Toss

Weight Loss Coconut Pudding

Cranberry & Broccoli Slaw

Spicy Onion & Fresh Mint Salsa

Low Carb Cauliflower Fillers

Broccoli Blasts

Fresh Coriander with Melons

Low Carb Celery Snack

Hot Chicken Paprika Wings

Egg & Parsley Evening Glee

Low Carb Spicy Egg & Coconut Salsa

Spicy Green Devilled Eggs

Hot Beef Quiche

Desserts Recipes

Almond with Lemon Fillings

Nuts & Pecan Desserts

Dried Dates Nuts Pie

Pecan with Pumpkin Feast

Nut Tart Berry Stuffs

High Protein Crust

Sugar Free Crust with Peach Stuffing

Macadamia with Berry Filling

Creamy Blueberry Filling

Sugar Free Carrot Bakes

Dried Chocolate Brown Cake

Rich Fruit Flax Dessert

Creamy Vanilla Scoop

Energy Reviving Almond Slices

Sugar Free Gingerly Pudding

Almond Vanilla Banana Pudding

Creamy Almond & Coconut Pie

New Yorkshire Pecan Chess Pies

Low Carb Almond & Cashew Balls

Baked Cranberries

Vanilla Coconut with Cashew Mascarpone

Very Berry Mixed Trifle

Vanilla Cocoa Almond Biscotti

Low Carb Wheat-Free Chocó Cake

Spicy Pumpkin Puree Cakes

Eating to Lose Weight!

Let's face it: many people could benefit from losing a few pounds. Indeed, just being slightly overweight can have a major influence on the risk of diabetes, stroke and heart disease. The statistics on obesity are alarming; CDC reports that over one-third of American adults are obese! This obesity trend is now affecting children, who are becoming increasingly overweight as well. Lack of physical activity along with poor food choices are the leading causes of this obesity epidemic. Sure, losing weight sounds easy in theory but not many people are willing to cut their calories and go hungry all day. Busy moms and dads don't always have time to do an hour of jogging every morning. So, what other options are there?

New research shows that counting fat grams or calories is not the best way to sustain a long-term weight loss. There are hundreds of fad diets that encourage people to starve themselves or eliminate an entire group of essential macronutrients (fat or carbohydrates) in order to lose a few pounds. You don't have to do this. The healthiest way to lose weight is to adopt a healthy lifestyle. While not necessarily the fastest weight loss plan, a healthy lifestyle can be adapted to your schedule and activities. What constitutes a healthy lifestyle varies from one person to another, but there are some general guidelines that can suit most people.

Convenience food is fantastic: buy a frozen pizza, turn on the over, do something else for 30 minutes and dinner is ready. Unfortunately, that frozen pizza is loaded with sugar, salt, unhealthy deli meats and preservatives. The overconsumption of foods that should be saved for special occasions is partly responsible for the obesity trend. Some people eat fast food, pizza, fried chicken or pastries on a daily basis While there is nothing wrong with these foods when consumed in moderation, they contribute to health problems when eaten every day.

Sugar is one of the top offenders when it comes to weight gain and health problems. Refined sugar is found in everything from sliced bread to sauces and hot dogs. Eliminating refined sugar and lowering overall sugar consumption is now thought to be one of the most important lifestyle changes for general health. Studies suggest that cutting out one can of soda per day and replacing it with plain water could lead to a 16 pound weight loss over a year with no other effort. Thus, cutting out soda entirely should be the first step to a healthy weight loss plan. If you've already eliminated soda from your diet, you can tackle the next step: processed ingredients and sugar in food.

Processing refers to the transformation of a product from its natural state to what you see on the grocery shelves. Fresh produce is generally unprocessed while frozen fruits and veggies bear minimal processing. Trouble starts with canned, bottled or boxed foods and frozen entrées. Manufacturers add liberal amounts of fat, sugar and salt to make these foods tasty. They strip the nutrients from grains in order to make baked goods with a better texture. They add preservatives, artificial flavors and MSG to nearly everything. Our bodies are not designed to eat these processed foods and respond with inflammation or disease.

Sugar is highly addictive. It makes things taste good and activates the release of happy hormones in the brain. When consumed on a regular basis, it leads to addiction, much like caffeine or nicotine. It also suppresses the release of hormones that signal a full stomach. The result is a craving to eat more food to fuel the addiction, and this urge is not suppressed by the natural hunger regulation mechanism.

Eliminating processed foods and sugar breaks this cycle. By making your own food at home, you can control exactly how much sweetener, salt and fat gets added. You will find yourself making better food choices, because you're actually giving some thought to what you put in your mouth. Studies have shown that weight tends to stabilize when on a healthy diet free of processed foods. It is indeed hard to overeat on veggies, eggs and meat because their high fiber or protein content triggers the necessary hormones that signal when enough food has been eaten.

To lose weight without counting calories or fat grams, make your own meals at home. Emphasize meat and vegetables, eggs and nuts, a little healthy fat such as olive or coconut oil, and add a couple of pieces of fruit.

Indulge in a glass of wine, a piece of dark chocolate or even a slice of cake once in a while. The key is to save these treats for special occasions. The weight should come off by itself. A slow and steady weight loss increases your chances of maintaining your target weight.

Adopting a whole new lifestyle can be challenging. This cookbook is designed to provide you with some delicious and healthy recipes to help you out on your weight loss journey. Each of these recipes features wholesome and healthy ingredients that are free of processed sugar and ingredients. Instead, a light touch of honey, date purée or stevia is used to enhance the taste. Processed white flour is eliminated; instead, crusts and doughs are made with hearty almond and coconut flours. White rice can be replaced with cauliflower "rice" and veggie spirals make great white pasta substitutes. When you eat real foods, you'll notice that you can eat until you are full and not worry about counting calories or carbs. Our modern lifestyle has stripped us of our ability to listen to our bodies, and regaining this ability is vital for healthy weight loss!

Foods to Avoid

You will want to avoid:

- White anything: white sugar, salt, bread, pasta, rice, flour, etc. These products are highly processed to remove all their nutrients, yielding a nutritionally dead "pure" product. Some companies enrich their white products to add a little nutrition back into these empty foods, but the overall difference is not that huge. Instead, opt for small portions of whole grains and limit your intake of these high-starch foods, since starch is also sugar.

- Commercial baked goods: they are almost always bad for you. Made with white flour, sugar and fat, there is much to be gained by baking them yourself.

- Sugar in all its forms: fructose, glucose solids, glucose-fructose, high-fructose corn syrup, corn syrup, evaporated cane juice, cane sugar, molasses, barley malt syrup, dextrose, isomalt and hundreds more. Use very small amounts of honey or stevia to lightly sweeten your baked treats.

- Artificial sweeteners: recent evidence suggests that artificial sweeteners increase weight gain by about 40%. Their metabolic effects are not very well-known and these should be avoided at all costs. The only acceptable no-calorie sweetener is stevia extract.

- Pre-packaged foods: sugar acts as a preservative and increases shelf life. Many canned veggies, pasta sauces, boxed dinners and frozen meals contain sugar or other unhealthy ingredients. Make a giant vegetable lasagna and freeze some leftovers for quick emergency dinners.

- Junk food and soda: there is very little place for these in a healthy diet. Save them for very special occasions, and be aware that they may trigger cravings for several days after consumption.

- Diet foods: any processed food marketed as fat-free, low-fat or low-calorie is probably high in something else such as sugar or artificial sweeteners. Avoid the low-fat salad dressings or the low-cal cranberry cocktails and make your own healthier versions.

Breakfast Ideas

Low Fat Seeds Feast

Prep Time: 10 minutes*

Servings: 2

INGREDIENTS

1/2 cup raw walnuts

1/2 cup raw almonds

1/4 cup raw pumpkin seeds

1/4 cup raw sunflower seeds

1/4 cup raw flax seeds

1 cup blueberries

1 cup raspberries

Vanilla Cream

1 cup raw cashews

2 tablespoons raw honey (or dried pitted dates)

1/2 teaspoon vanilla

1/8 teaspoon Celtic sea salt

Water

INSTRUCTIONS

1. *Soak cashews and dates (if using) in enough water to cover at least 6 hours, or overnight in refrigerator. Drain and set aside.
2. Add walnuts, almonds, pumpkin, sunflower and flax seeds to food processor or high-speed blender. Pulse to coarsely chop. Set aside.
3. For *Vanilla Cream*, add soaked cashews, honey or dates, vanilla and salt to clean food processor or high-speed blender. Process

until smooth, about 1 - 2 minutes. Add enough water or nut milk to reach desired consistency.

4. Spoon layer of fruit into serving dish. Top with chopped nuts. Spoon on layer of *Vanilla Cream*. Add second layer of chopped nuts. Top with layer of fruit.

5. Serve immediately. Or refrigerate 20 minutes and serve chilled.

Weight Loss Whole Chia Pudding

Prep Time: 10 minutes*

Servings: 2

INGREDIENTS

2 coconuts (or 1 cup flaked coconut)

6 dried pitted dates

3 tablespoons whole chia seeds

2 tablespoons cocoa powder

1/2 teaspoon vanilla

1/2 teaspoon ground black pepper

Pinch cayenne pepper

Pinch chili powder

Pinch smoked paprika

Water

INSTRUCTIONS

1. *Soak flaked coconut in 2 cups water overnight in refrigerator, if using. Soak dates in enough water to cover at least 4 hours, or overnight in refrigerator. Drain dates.
2. Add soaked coconut and soaking liquid to high-speed blender. Or remove flesh from fresh coconuts and add to high-speed blender with 2 cups water. Process until well blended and fairly smooth, about 1 - 2 minutes.
3. Strain mixture through nut milk bag, cheesecloth or strainer back into blender.

4. Reserve pulp and set aside to dry and dehydrate, then use as coconut flour.
5. Add dates, cocoa, vanilla and spices to blender. Process until smooth, about 1 minute.
6. Pour mixture into serving dish and stir in chia seeds. Set aside to thicken, about 1 minute.
7. Serve immediately. Or refrigerate 20 minutes and serve chilled.

Sugar Free Chia Pudding

Prep Time: 10 minutes*

Servings: 2

INGREDIENTS

2 coconuts (or 1 cup flaked coconut)

2 - 4 tablespoons raw honey (or dried pitted dates)

1/4 cup tablespoons whole chia seeds

1 cup strawberries (fresh or frozen and thawed, chopped)

1/2 teaspoon vanilla

Water

INSTRUCTIONS

1. *Soak flaked coconut in 2 cups water overnight in refrigerator, if using. Soak dates in enough water to cover at least 4 hours, or overnight in refrigerator, if using. Drain dates.

2. Add soaked coconut and soaking liquid to high-speed blender. Or remove flesh from fresh coconuts and add to high-speed blender with 2 cups water. Process until well blended and fairly smooth, about 1 - 2 minutes.

3. Strain mixture through nut milk bag, cheesecloth or strainer back into blender.

4. Reserve pulp and set aside to dry and dehydrate, then use as coconut flour.

5. Remove stems from strawberries, then cut in half. Add to blender with honey or dates, and vanilla. Process until smooth, about 1 minute.

6. Pour mixture into serving dish and stir in chia seeds. Set aside to thicken, about 1 minute.

7. Serve immediately. Or refrigerate 20 minutes and serve chilled.

Rich Nuts Blend

Prep Time: 10 minutes

Servings: 2

INGREDIENTS

1 coconut (1/2 cup flaked coconut)

3/4 cup raw nuts (any combination of cashews, almonds, brazil nuts, acorns, macadamia nuts, etc.)

2 overripe bananas

2 teaspoons ground cinnamon

1/4 teaspoon vanilla

1/4 teaspoon Celtic sea salt

Water

INSTRUCTIONS

1. * Soak nuts in enough water to cover for at least 6 hours, or overnight in refrigerator. Drain and rinse, then set aside. Soak flaked coconut in 2 cups water in refrigerator overnight, if using.

2. Add soaked coconut and soaking liquid to high-speed blender. Or remove flesh from fresh coconut and add to high-speed blender with 2 cups water. Process until well blended and fairly smooth, about 1 - 2 minutes.

3. Strain mixture through nut milk bag, cheesecloth or strainer back into blender or food processor.

4. Reserve pulp and set aside to dry and dehydrate, then use as coconut flour.

5. Peel bananas and add to processor with vanilla, salt and 1 teaspoon cinnamon. Process until thick and mostly smooth, about 1 minute.

6. Transfer to serving dish and serve immediately.

Tangy Carrot Salad

Prep Time: 5 minutes

Servings: 1

INSTRUCTIONS

2 large carrots

3 tablespoon dried cranberries

1/4 cup raw almonds

1/2 small orange (or tangerine)

1/2 piece fresh ginger

1/2 teaspoon ground ginger

DIRECTIONS

1. Add carrots to food processor with shredding attachment and process, or grate with grater. Add to medium mixing bowl with cranberries and ground ginger.

2. Add almonds to food processor and pulse to coarsely chop. Or add to paper or plastic kitchen bag and pound with heavy rolling pin to crush. Peel ginger and dice or finely grate. Zest *then* juice orange. Add to carrot mixture and toss to combine.

3. Transfer to serving dish and serve immediately. Or refrigerate 20 minutes and serve chilled.

Easy Fruit Salad

Prep Time: 5 minutes

Servings: 1

INSTRUCTIONS

1 apple

1 small banana

1/4 cup blueberries

1/4 cup raw almonds

2 dried pitted dates

2 tablespoons pomegranate seeds (or dried goji or noni berries)

1/4 teaspoon ground cinnamon

INGREDIENTS

1. Core and dice apple. Peel and dice banana. Add to serving dish and mix to combine. Top with blueberries.
2. Chop almonds and dates. Or add to food processor and pulse to coarsely grind.
3. Top fruit with chopped nuts and dates. Sprinkle with pomegranate seeds and cinnamon and serve immediately.

Morning Berry Dish

Prep Time: 10 minutes

Servings: 1

INSTRUCTIONS

1 nectarine

1/2 cup strawberries

1/4 cup blackberries

1/4 cup blueberry

1/4 cup cherries

1/4 cup raw nuts (cashews, almonds, brazil nuts, acorns, macadamia, etc.)

1/2 inch piece fresh ginger

Small sprig fresh mint

INGREDIENTS

1. Cut nectarine in half and remove pit. Dice and add to small mixing bowl. Remove stems from strawberries and quarter. Pit cherries. Add to bowl with blackberries and blueberries.

2. Peel ginger and mince or finely grate. Chiffon mint leaves. Add to bowl and toss to combine. Transfer to serving dish.

3. Add nuts to food processor and pulse to coarsely chop. Or add to paper or plastic kitchen bag and pound with heavy rolling pin to crush.

4. Sprinkle on nuts and serve immediately. Or refrigerate 20 minutes and serve chilled.

Sugar Free Low Fat Salad

Prep Time: 10 minutes

Servings: 1

INSTRUCTIONS

1 fresh coconut (or 1/2 cup flaked coconut)

1/4 - 1/3 cup dried pitted dates (or raw honey)

1 blood orange

1 tangerine (or navel orange or clementine)

1/2 grapefruit (ruby red, pink or white)

1/2 lime

1 tablespoon sunflower seeds (optional)

Water

INGREDIENTS

1. *Soak flaked coconut in 1 cup water overnight in refrigerator, if using. Soak dates in enough water to cover overnight in refrigerator. Drain.

2. Add soaked coconut and soaking liquid to high-speed blender. Or remove flesh from fresh coconut and add to high-speed blender with 3/4 cup water. Process until thick and fairly smooth, about 1 - 2 minutes.

3. Strain mixture through nut milk bag, cheesecloth or strainer back into blender or to food processor.

4. Reserve pulp and set aside to dry and dehydrate, then use as coconut flour.

5. Add soaked dates or honey to processor and process until smooth. Set aside.
6. Peel all citrus and cut into segments. Add to serving dish. Top with sweet coconut cream. Sprinkle on sunflower seeds (optional).
7. Serve immediately. Or refrigerate 20 minutes and serve chilled.

Ground Dice

Prep Time: 5 minutes

Servings: 1

INGREDIENTS

2 ripe peaches (or nectarines)

4 dried pitted dates

1/3 cup raw almonds

1/4 teaspoon ground cinnamon

1/4 teaspoon ground ginger

1/8 teaspoon vanilla

1/8 teaspoon ground white pepper (or ground black pepper)

INSTRUCTIONS

1. Add dates, almonds vanilla and spices to food processor or high-speed blender. Pulse to coarsely grind, about 1 minute.
2. Cut peaches in half and remove pits. Dice peaches and transfer to serving dish.
3. Sprinkle on almond mixture and serve immediately.

Low Fat Berry Breakfast

Prep Time: 5 minutes*

Servings: 1

INGREDIENTS

1 1/2 cups raw cashews

1 banana

1/4 cup blueberries

1 tablespoon raw honey (or 2 pitted dates)

1 tablespoon lemon juice

1/4 teaspoon vanilla

1/4 teaspoon Celtic sea salt

Water

INSTRUCTIONS

1. *Soak cashews and dates (if using) in enough water to cover overnight in refrigerator. Drain.
2. Peel banana. Add to food processor or high-speed blender with soaked cashews, dates or honey, lemon juice, vanilla and salt. Process until thick and fairly smooth, about 1 - 2 minutes. Add enough water to reach desired consistency.
3. Transfer to serving dish and top with blueberries. Serve immediately.

Vanilla Nuts Meal

Prep Time: 10 minutes*

Servings: 1

INGREDIENTS

3/4 cup raw almonds

1/3 cups raw walnuts

1/3 cups cashews

1/4 cup raw pumpkin seeds

1/4 cup shredded or flaked coconut

2 tablespoon dried cranberries

1/3 cup dried pitted dates

1/4 tablespoon vanilla

1/4 tablespoon cinnamon

1/4 teaspoon ground ginger

1/2 teaspoon Celtic sea salt

Water

INSTRUCTIONS

1. *Separately soak 1/4 cup almonds in enough water to cover at least 6 hours, or overnight. Drain and rinse. Soak 1/4 cupdates in enough water to cover at least 6 hours, or overnight. Drain.

2. Add soaked almonds to high-speed blender with 2/3 - 3/4 cup water. Process until well blended and almost smooth, about 1- 2 minutes.

3. Strain mixture through nut milk bag, cheesecloth or strainer back into blender.

4. Add soaked dates to blender with vanilla, salt and ginger. Process until smooth, about 1 minutes. Add to medium mixing bowl.
5. Chop remaining almonds, walnuts and dates by hand. Or add to clean food processor or high-speed blender and pulse to roughly chop. Add to bowl with pumpkin seeds, flaked coconut, cranberries and cinnamon. Mix to combine.
6. Transfer to serving dish and serve immediately. Or refrigerate 20 minutes and serve chilled.

Low Fat Goji Flax Bowl

Prep Time: 5 minutes*

Servings: 2

INGREDIENTS

2 cage free eggs (optional)

1/2 apple

1/4 cup flaked or shredded coconut

1/4 - 1/3 cup dried pitted dates

1/3 cup raw walnuts

1/3 cup raw almonds

2 tablespoons coconut oil (or coconut butter or cacao butter)

2 tablespoons flax seed (or chia seed)

2 tablespoons raisins

2 tablespoons dried goji berries (optional)

1 teaspoon ground cinnamon

Pinch Celtic sea salt

Water

INSTRUCTIONS

1. *Soak walnuts and almonds in enough water to cover for at least 6 hours, or overnight in refrigerator. Drain and rinse, then set aside. Soak dates in enough water to cover for at least 6 hours, or overnight in refrigerator. Drain and set aside. Soak flaked coconut in 1 cup water overnight in refrigerator.

2. Add flax or chia to food processor or high-speed blender and process until finely ground. Add coconut oil and process until thick paste forms.
3. Add dates, nuts, eggs, cinnamon, salt, soaked coconut and soaking liquid to processor. Process until thick mixture forms, about 1 - 2 minutes. Transfer to serving dish.
4. Core and dice apple. Top with dices apple, raisins and goji berries (optional).
5. Serve immediately.

Nut Cakes

Prep Time: 15 minutes*

Dehydrating Time: 8 - 9 hours

Servings: 2

INGREDIENTS

Pancakes

1 young coconut (plus coconut water)

1/2 cup raw cashews (or 1/4 cup raw cashew butter)

1/4 cup flax seed

1/4 teaspoon ground cinnamon

1/2 teaspoon vanilla

Water

Berry Jam

1 orange

1/4 cup dried raspberries

1/4 cup dried cherries

1/4 cup dried strawberries

 Water

INSTRUCTIONS

1. *Soak dried fruit in enough water to cover at least 4 hours, or overnight in refrigerator. Drain and reserve soaking liquid. Set aside.

2. For *Pancakes*, add flax to food processor or high-speed blender. Process until finely ground, about 2 minutes.

3. Add cashews to processor, if using. Process until smooth, up to 5 minutes. Or use prepared cashew butter.

4. Remove flesh and water from young coconut add and add to processor with cashew butter, cinnamon and vanilla cardamom. Process until smooth batter forms, about 1 - 2 minutes. Add enough water to reach desired consistency.

5. Place parchment paper or dehydrator sheets on dehydrator trays.

6. Use spoon to spread batter on prepared sheets in 2 x 2 inch circles 1/4 inch thick. Place trays in dehydrator and set to 110 degrees F for 6 hours.

7. Remove trays from dehydrator. Flip *Pancakes* and place trays back in dehydrator. Continue dehydrating 2 - 3 hours, until surface is dry but *Pancakes* are still moist and pliable.

8. For *Berry Jam*, zest *then* juice orange into clean food processor or high-speed blender. Add soaked fruit and process until mostly smooth, about 1 minute. Add enough soaking liquid and/or water to reach desired consistency and sweetness.

9. Remove *Pancakes* from dehydrator and transfer to serving dish. Top with *Berry Jam* and serve immediately.

Creamy Coconut Breakfast

Prep Time: 10 minutes*

Servings: 2

INGREDIENTS

Coconut Breakfast Cake

1 fresh coconut (or 1/2 cup flaked or shredded coconut)

1/2 cup ground flax seed (or chia seed)

1/4 cup raw honey (or 1/3 cup dried pitted dates)

2 tablespoons coconut oil (or coconut butter or cacao butter)

1/2 teaspoon ground cinnamon

1/4 teaspoon Celtic sea salt

Water

Apricot Jam

1 cup dried apricots

2 tablespoons lemon juice

1/4 inch piece fresh ginger (or 1/2 teaspoon ground ginger)

Water

INSTRUCTIONS

1. *For *Coconut Breakfast Cakes*, soak flaked coconut and in 1 cup water overnight in refrigerator, if using. Soak dates in enough water to cover overnight in refrigerator, if using. Drain.

2. Add soaked coconut and soaking liquid to high-speed blender. Or remove flesh from fresh coconut and add to high-speed blender with 1 cup water, ground flax or chia, soaked dates or honey,

coconut oil, salt and cinnamon. Pulse to coarsely grind, until mixture sticks together.

3. Form mixture into 6 balls and flatten into cakes. Or mold in lined muffin tins. Set aside.

4. For *Apricot Jam*, peel ginger and add to clean food processor or high-speed blender with apricots and lemon juice. Process until smooth, about 1 minute. Add enough water to reach desired consistency.

5. Transfer *Coconut Breakfast Cakes* to serving dish. Top with *Apricot Jam* and serve immediately. Or refrigerate 20 minutes and serve chilled.

Easy Weight Loss Almond Teaser

Prep Time: 5 minutes

Cook Time: 20 minutes

Servings: 4

INGREDIENTS

1 cup almond flour

1/4 cup ground chia seed (or flax seed meal)

1 tablespoon vanilla

1 teaspoon ground nutmeg

1 teaspoon ground cinnamon

1/2 cup raw agave nectar (or 1/2 cup raw honey + 1 tablespoon water)

1 cup flakedcoconut

1 cup sliced almonds

1/2 cup dried figs

1/2 cup dried dates

1/2 cup pecans

1/2 cup pumpkin seeds

1/2 cup dried apricots

1/2 cup coconut oil, melted

INSTRUCTIONS

1. Preheat oven to 350 degrees F. Lightly coat cookie sheet with coconut oil.
2. Stem figs and pit dates. Chop figs, dates, pecans and apricots. Add to medium bowl, along with all other ingredients. Mix to combine, then spread evenly over sheet pan with spatula.

3. Bake in preheated oven for about 10 minutes. Then carefully remove and use spatula to turn over par-baked granola. Bake for additional8 -10 minutes. Check periodically to ensure nuts do not over-toast.
4. Remove from oven and let cool and firm. Serve cool.

Almond Meal Vanilla Pancakes

Prep Time: 5 minutes

Cook Time: 15 minutes

Servings: 2

INGREDIENTS

1 3/4 cups almond meal

2 eggs

3/4 cup almond milk

2 medium carrots

1/4 cup chopped walnuts

1/4 cup golden raisins (optional)

1 teaspoon baking powder

1 tablespoon ground cinnamon

1 teaspoon ground nutmeg

1 teaspoon ground ginger

1 teaspoon vanilla

1/4 teaspoon sea salt

Pinch of ground black pepper

INSTRUCTIONS

1. Heat large skillet on medium-high heat and lightly coat with oil.
2. Finely grate carrots and drain in paper towel, or roughly process in food processor or bullet blender.
3. In medium bowl whisk eggs, almond milk, vanilla, cinnamon, nutmeg, ginger and black pepper.

4. Add almond flour, salt and baking powder. Whisk until smooth. Stir in carrots, walnuts and raisins (optional).

5. Use ladle or dry measure cup to pour 1/3 cup of batter onto hot oiled skillet. Fit 2 or 3 pancakes comfortably, so they do not touch as they spread.

6. Cook until sides of pancakes are firm and batter bubbles up a bit. About 3 - 4 minutes.

7. Carefully flip pancakes with spatula and cook for additional minute, or until cooked through. Repeat with remaining batter. Re-oil pan if necessary. Pancakes will be slightly delicate, so flip and plate with care.

8. Serve warm. Sprinkle with cinnamon and drizzle with agave nectar, or topping of choice.

Ground Flax Seed Breakfast Burrito

Prep Time: 10 minutes

Cook Time: 10 minutes

Servings: 2

INGREDIENTS

Tortillas:

2 tablespoons coconut flour

2 tablespoons almond flour

2 teaspoons ground flax seed

2 eggs

2 tablespoons melted coconut oil

1/4 teaspoon baking powder

1/4 - 1/2 cup water

Coconut oil (for cooking)

Filling:

6 oz natural pre-cooked ham

6 eggs

1 bell pepper

1/2 red onion

1 avocado

4 oz organic salsa

Pinch sea salt

Pinch ground black pepper

INSTRUCTIONS

1. Heat largepan over medium-high heat and coat with 2 tablespoons of coconut oil. Heat second skillet over medium heat and lightly coat with coconut oil.

2. For **Tortillas**, blend coconut flour, almond flour, flax meal and baking powder in medium bowl. In separate bowl, whisk together 2 eggs, 2 tablespoons coconut oil and 1/4 cup water.

3. Slowly whisk dry blend into wet mixture. Whisk as you pour to avoid clumps. Continue to whisk and slowly add just enough water to make thin but hearty batter.

4. Once coconut oil is hot, use ladle or dry measure cup to pour half of batter into large pan. Tilt pan in circular motion as you pour so batter spreads thinly.Cook batter for about 2 minutes or until tortilla is slightly golden and firm.

5. While **Tortillas** cook, seed and stem pepper and peel onion. Chop ham, pepper and onion. Add to second skillet and sauté for about 2 minutes.

6. Flip tortilla and cook for 2 more minutes. Remove when toasted and cooked through. Place on paper towel or parchment. Add remaining batter to large pan, repeating tilting process to create thin tortilla.

7. While second tortilla cooks , beat 6 eggs in medium bowl and pour over veggies and ham. Salt and pepper to taste. Scramble until desired firmness.

8. Fill both tortillas down center each with half of ham scramble. Slice avocado in half, pit,then scoop out flesh onto each burrito.

9. Roll up tortillas and plate fold-side down. Dollop with your favorite salsa. Serve warm.

Coconut Flour Breakfast Pizza

Prep Time: 10 minutes

Cook Time: 15 minutes

Servings: 2

INGREDIENTS

Crust:

1 1/2 cup almond flour

1/4 cup tablespoons coconut flour

2 eggs

1 tablespoon melted coconut oil

Coconut oil (for cooking)

Topping:

4 eggs

4 oz pre-cooked natural sausage

1/2 small red onions

1 /2 green pepper

1 whole roasted red pepper (jarred)

Handful black olives

1 tablespoon rosemary

Pinch ground black pepper

Pinch sea salt

INSTRUCTIONS

1. Preheat oven to 425 degrees F. Heat medium skillet to medium heat and lightly coat with coconut oil. Coat 8 or 9-inch round cake pan with coconut oil and dust with coconut flour.

2. Combine all *Crust* ingredients in small bowl. If too soft, add 1 tablespoon of coconut flour at a time. If too firm, add 1 tablespoon of water at a time. Adjust until firm dough that can hold its shape forms.

3. Form dough into ball and place in cake pan. Gently pat it into 1/4 inch thick circle, building up around edge about 1/2 - 1 inch up sides of pan. Bake crust for 5 minutes.

4. Chop sausage and rosemary. Seed and stem green pepper and peel onion. Slice onion and pepper and add to skillet with sausage. Sauté about 2 minutes.

5. Whisk eggs in medium bowl and add eggs to skillet, plus rosemary. Remove skillet from heat and scramble very lightly.

6. Reduce oven to 350 degrees F and remove pan.Carefully pour runny scrambled eggs into crust. Slice roasted red pepper and olives and sprinkle over eggs. Salt and pepper to taste.

7. Return pizza to oven and bake another 10 - 15 minutes or until eggs firm.

8. Slice and serve hot from pan. Or remove, slice and serve.

Low Carb Romaine Lettuce Salad

Prep Time: 10 minutes

Cook Time: 5 minutes

Servings: 1

INGREDIENTS

Salad:

4 slices turkey bacon

1 tablespoon coconut oil

1 heart of romaine lettuce

2medium tomatoes, chopped

Dressing:

1 avocado

1/2 small white onion

1 small garlic clove

Juice of 1 lemon

Small bunch of parsley leaves

Pinch sea salt

Pinch ground black pepper

INSTRUCTIONS

1. Heat medium skillet to medium-high heat and add coconut oil.
2. Chop turkey bacon and add to skillet. Browned for 2 - 3 minutes on each side, until thoroughly cooked. Remove turkey bacon and preserve any leftover oil.

3. Rinse and dry heart of romaine, then chop. Dice tomato and toss with lettuce in large bowl.

4. For **Dressing**, slice avocado in half, pit, and spoon flesh into food processor or bullet blender. Add peeled onion and garlic, lemon juice and parsley. Add excess coconut oil from pan.Process until smooth. Salt and pepper to taste.

5. Use tongs to transfer lettuce and tomatoes to plate. Sprinkle on turkey bacon, and drizzle with avocado **Dressing**. Serve immediately.

Chia Seed Dates Oatmeal

Prep Time: 5 minutes

Cook Time: 10 minutes

Servings: 2

INGREDIENTS

2 cups coconut milk

1/2 cup quick tapioca

1/4 cup chia seed

1/2 cup dried dates

1 small banana

2 tablespoons slivered almonds

2 tablespoons pumpkin seeds

2 tablespoons flaked coconut

2 tablespoons walnuts

1 tablespoon vanilla

1 teaspoon ground cinnamon

2 tablespoons raw agave nectar (optional)

Pinch sea salt

Water

INSTRUCTIONS

1. Heat medium pan over medium heat .
2. Add almonds, pumpkin seeds, coconut flakes and walnuts to hot dry pan. Dry toast about 2 minutes, stirring frequently to prevent burning.

3. Pit and chop dates. Cut banana in half and blend with coconut milk and dates in food processor or bullet blender. Reserve other half of banana.

4. Add milk mixture to hot pan. Add quick tapioca, chia seeds, vanilla and pinch of salt. Stir and thicken over heat about 5 - 8 minutes, or until tapioca is soft. Add water to loosen for runnier "oatmeal."

5. Slice reserved half of banana. Serve hot in bowl. Top with banana slices, sprinkle with cinnamon, and drizzle with agave (optional).

Spicy Almond Meal

Prep Time: 5 minutes

Cook Time: 15 minutes

Servings: 2

INGREDIENTS

Pancakes:

1 3/4 cups almond meal

3/4 cup almond milk

2 eggs

1 teaspoon baking powder

1 teaspoon vanilla

Pinch sea salt

Pinch ground black pepper

Agave nectar (optional)

Coconut oil (for cooking)

Filling:

4 eggs

INSTRUCTIONS

1. Heat large skillet with lid over medium heat and lightly coat with coconut oil.

2. Whisk together 2 eggs, almond milk and vanilla in medium bowl. Whisk in almond flour, baking powder and salt until smooth.

3. Use ladle or dry measure cup to pour 1/3 of batter onto hot oiled skillet in a circle with a hole large enough for one egg. Fit up to 2 pancakes comfortably, so they do not touch as they spread.

4. Crack one egg into each space within pancake. Cover with lid and cook until sides of pancakes are firm and batter bubbles up a bit. About 3 - 4 minutes.

5. Remove lid and gently flip pancakes with spatula, careful to keep yolks intact. Cookuncovered for about 3 minutes, or until pancakesarecooked through.

6. Repeat with remaining batter. Re-oil pan if necessary. Pancakes will be slightly delicate, so flip and plate with care.

7. Sprinkle egg with salt and pepper to taste. Drizzle with agave nectar (optional). Serve warm.

Spicy Bacon With Egg Scramble

Prep Time: 10 minutes

Cook Time: 15 minutes

Servings: 2

INGREDIENTS

6 eggs

4 slices nitrate-free bacon

2 dried figs

1 sweet apple

1 bell pepper

1 small sweet onion

1/2 teaspoon ground black pepper

1/2 teaspoon paprika

1/2teaspoon sea salt

1/2 teaspoon cinnamon (optional)

INSTRUCTIONS

1. Bring small pot to boil with lightly salted water. Heat medium skillet over medium-high heat.
2. Dice bacon and add to hot skillet. Brown bacon for about 3 minutes, stirring occasionally with wooden spatula.
3. Add figs to boiling water for 5 minutes.
4. Peel and core apple. Stem and seed pepper. Peel onion. Dice apple, pepper and onion and add to skillet. Sauté another 2 minutes, until veggies caramelize and bacon crisps.

5. Remove figs from boiling water and dice. Add to skillet, plus spices. Sauté another minute.

6. Crack eggs directly into skillet and scramble gently with wooden spatula.

7. Cook eggs to desired firmness and serve hot.

Egg with Pork Sausage Breakfast Skillet

Prep Time: 5 minutes

Cook Time: 15 minutes

Servings: 2

INGREDIENTS

6 eggs

8 oz ground pork sausage

1 medium sweet potato

1 bell pepper

1 small red onion

Ground black pepper, to taste

Paprika, to taste

sea salt, to taste

Pinch of cinnamon (optional)

INSTRUCTIONS

1. Bring medium pot to boil with lightly salted water. Leave enough room in pot for sweet potato. Heat large skillet over medium-high heat.

2. Peel and dice sweet potato. Add to boiling water for 5 minutes.

3. Add sausage to hot skillet. Brown sausage for 5 minutes, stirring occasionally with wooden spatula.

4. While potatoes and sausage cook, seed and vein bell pepper and peel onion, then dice.

5. Beat eggs with spices in medium bowl with hand mixer or whisk.

6. Once browned, add pepper and onion to sausage. Sauté about 2 minutes, until vegetables are tender and a bit caramelized.
7. Drain sweet potatoes in colander and add to skillet. Sauté about 1 minute, until any excess liquid is evaporated. Then pour in egg mixture.
8. Scramble eggs with wooden spatula. Reduce skillet to medium heat to cook eggs evenly and avoid browning.
9. Cook and stir eggs until desired firmness. Remove from heat and serve.

Almond Meal Banana Pancakes

Prep Time: 5 minutes

Cook Time: 15 minutes

Servings: 2

INGREDIENTS

Pancakes:

1 3/4 cups almond meal

1 teaspoon baking powder

2 eggs

3/4 cup coconut milk

1/4 cup flaked coconut

1/2 banana

1 teaspoon vanilla

1/4 teaspoon sea salt

Coconut oil (for cooking)

Topping:

1/2 banana

Agave nectar (optional)

INSTRUCTIONS

1. Heat a large skillet over medium-high heat and lightly coat with coconut oil.
2. Mash 1/2 banana in medium bowl with fork. Whisk in eggs, then coconut milk and vanilla.

3. Add almond flour, salt and baking powder. Whisk until smooth. Fold in coconut flakes.

4. Use ladle or dry measure cup to pour 1/4 cup of batter onto hot oiled skillet. Fit 2 or 3 pancakes comfortably, so they do not touch as they spread.

5. Cook until sides of pancakes are firm and batter bubbles up a bit. About 3 to 4 minutes.

6. Carefully flip pancakes with spatula and cook for additional minute, or until cooked through. Repeat with remaining batter. Re-oil pan if necessary. Pancakes will be slightly delicate, so flip and plate with care.

7. Slice 1/2 banana. Top with banana slices and agave nectar. Serve warm.

Cinnamon & Pumpkin with Bacon Treat

Prep Time: 5 minutes

Cook Time: 15 minutes

Servings: 2

INGREDIENTS

1 3/4 cups almond flour

1 cup almond milk

1/2 cup pumpkin puree

2 eggs

1 teaspoon baking powder

2 teaspoons ground cinnamon

1 teaspoon vanilla

1/4 teaspoon sea salt

4 slices nitrate-free bacon

INSTRUCTIONS

1. Heat large skillet over high heat.
2. Chop bacon into 1/2 inch pieces. Add to hot skillet and brown. Stir occasionally with wooden spoon.
3. Whisk eggs in medium bowl. Then whisk in almond milk, pumpkin puree, vanilla and cinnamon.
4. Add almond flour, salt and baking powder. Whisk until smooth.
5. Once crisp, reduce pan to medium heat and remove bacon from pan, leaving drippings. Drain bacon bits on paper towel, then stir into pancake mixture.

6. Use ladle or dry measure cup to pour 1/4 cup of batter onto hot oiled skillet. Fit 2 or 3 pancakes comfortably, so they do not touch as they spread.

7. Cook until sides of pancakes are firm and batter bubbles up a bit. About 3 to 4 minutes.

8. Carefully flip pancakes with spatula and cook for additional minute, or until cooked through. Repeat with remaining batter. Pancakes will be slightly delicate, so flip and plate with care.

Serve warm. Top with topping of choice.

Easy Lunch Recipes

Low Fat Skinless Chicken Flax Meal

Prep Time: 10 minutes

Cook Time: 15 minutes

Servings: 2

INGREDIENTS

8 oz boneless, skinless chicken breast

1 egg

1/2 cup almond meal

1 teaspoon flax meal (or ground chia seed)

1 teaspoon ground black pepper

1/2 teaspoon paprika

1/2 teaspoon onion powder

1/2 teaspoon garlic powder

1/2 teaspoon chili powder

1/2 teaspoon sea salt

Garlic Aioli

1/2 - 3/4 cup coconut oil

1 egg yolk

2 garlic cloves

1/2 small lemon

1/4 teaspoon ground white pepper (or black pepper)

1/4 teaspoon sea salt

3 tablespoons flavorful oil (black truffle, walnut, almond, sesame, etc.)
(optional)

INSTRUCTIONS

1. Heat large pan over medium-high heat and coat with coconut oil.

2. For *Garlic Aioli*, peel garlic and add to food processor or blender with egg yolk, juice of 1/2 lemon, salt and pepper. Process until smooth, scraping down sides of vessel.

3. While processor or blender is running, very slowly drizzle in enough coconut oil to create thick mayo-like mixture. Drizzle in flavorful oil as well will processor runs (optional). If mixture is runny, drizzle in more coconut oil while processor runs until thickened. Pour into serving dish and refrigerate.

4. Slice chicken into half width-wise, creating twice the fillets. Try to slice at thickest portion to keep all fillets equal thickness.

5. Slice chicken fillets into long, 1/2 inch wide strips. Place strips between two paper towels and press to absorb excess moisture.

6. In a shallow dish, blend almond meal, flax or chia meal, spices and salt.

7. Beat egg in small mixing bowl. Toss chicken strips in beaten egg to lightly coat, then dredge in seasoned almond meal.

8. Carefully place coated chicken strips into hot oil and fry about 2 - 3minutes, until golden brown and cooked through. Turn with tongs half way through cooking.

9. Drain cooked chicken on paper towel, then transfer to serving dish.

10. Serve hot with *Garlic Aioli*.

Tuna Sandwich

Prep Time: 10 minutes

Cook Time: 15 minutes

Servings: 1

INSTRUCTIONS

Sandwich Bread

7oz (1 can) chunk light tuna

1/2 avocado

1/2 small red onion

1 small carrot

1 small celery stalk

1/2 small cucumber

1/2 lemon

1/2 teaspoon paprika

1/4 teaspoon cracked black pepper (or ground black pepper)

1/4 teaspoon sea salt

DIRECTIONS

1. Preheat oven to 350 degrees F. Lightly coat 6 mini round cake pans or medium loaf pan with coconut oil. Bring medium pot of lightly salted water to a boil.
2. Prepare *Sandwich Bread* and place in oven.
3. While bread bakes, drain tuna and add to small mixing bowl. Cut celery stalk and carrot in half length-wise. Peel onion and cucumber. Finely dice celery, carrot and onion. Add to bowl.

4. Slice avocado in half and scoop flesh of non-pit half into bowl. Preserve pitted half in airtight container with pit intact for freshness.
5. Add salt, pepper paprika and squeeze of 1/2 lemon into bowl. Mash together with fork until combined and smooth. Slice cucumber into 1/4 inch rounds.
6. Refrigerate tuna mixture if preferred.
7. Remove *Sandwich Bread* from oven and let cool about 5 minutes.
8. Slice bread and fill with tuna mixture. Top with cucumber slices.
9. Serve immediately.

Low Fat Chicken Cauliflower Slices

Prep Time: 10 minutes

Cook Time: 15 minutes

Servings: 4

INGREDIENTS

1 head cauliflower

8 oz boneless, skinless chicken

1 mango

1 hot chili pepper

2 scallions

2 garlic cloves

3 tablespoons pure fish sauce (or coconut aminos)

3 teaspoons sesame oil (or walnut or almond oil)

1/2 teaspoon red pepper flake

1/2 lime

Coconut oil (for cooking)

INSTRUCTIONS

1. Heat large skillet or medium cast-iron wok over high heat. Lightly coat with coconut oil.

2. Cut cauliflower into florets and add to food processor with shredding attachment to rice. Or finely mince cauliflower.

3. Peel garlic and ginger and mince. Mince chili pepper. Thinly slice scallions. Carefully peel and dice mango. Dice chicken.

4. Add diced chicken, garlic, ginger, chili pepper and red pepper flake to hot skillet or wok. Sauté until chicken is golden brown and just cooked, about 3 minutes. Remove chicken and set aside.

5. Add cauliflower to hot pan or wok. Sauté about 5 minutes, until cauliflower is golden and a bit softened.

6. Add mango and scallions and cook another 2 - 5minutes, until cauliflower is cooked through.

7. Add chicken to cauliflower and stir.

8. Remove from heat and serve hot with a squeeze of lime.

Ground Beef Mexican Oregano Fry

Prep Time: 5 minutes

Cook Time: 20 minutes

Servings: 4

INGREDIENTS

1 lb lean grass-fed ground beef (or elk, bison, turkey or chicken)

15 oz (1 can) organic tomato sauce

6oz (1 can) organic tomato paste

1 small onion

1 bell pepper

2 cloves garlic

2 tablespoons chili powder

1 tablespoon ground cumin

1 tablespoon smoked paprika (or paprika)

1 teaspoon Mexican oregano (or dried oregano)

1 teaspoon ground black pepper

1 teaspoon sea salt

1/2 teaspoon cayenne pepper

1 tablespoon coconut oil

sea salt, to taste

INSTRUCTIONS

1. Heat medium pot over medium-high heat. Add 1 tablespoon coconut oil.

2. Peel onion and garlic. Stem and seed bell pepper. Chop and add to food processor or bullet blender. Pulse until finely minced.

3. Add to skillet and sauté for about 1 minute. Add ground beef and spices. Brown beef for about 5 minutes. Stir with whisk to break up meat well, or wooden spoon to keep beef chunkier.

4. Add whole cans of tomato sauce and paste. Stir to combine.

5. Bring to a simmer, then reduce heat to medium and cover loosely with lid to prevent splatter. Simmer about 10 minutes. Stir occasionally.

6. Use large serving spoon or ladle to serve hot.

Almond Creamy Cakes

Prep Time: 5 minutes

Cook Time: 15 minutes

Servings: 6

INGREDIENTS

1/4 cup almond flour

1/4 cup coconut flour

4 eggs

2 tablespoons coconut oil

2 tablespoons unsweetened applesauce

1 teaspoon flax meal (or ground chia seed)

1 teaspoon baking powder

1/2 teaspoon sea salt

INSTRUCTIONS

1. Preheat oven to 350 degrees F. Line sheet pan with parchment paper, or lightly coat with coconut oil. Or lightly coat 6 mini round cake pans with coconut oil.

2. Beat eggs, coconut oil and applesauce in medium mixing bowl with hand mixer or whisk.

3. In large mixing bowl, sift together coconut flour, almond flour, flax or chia meal, baking powder and salt. Pour egg mixture into flour mixture and mix until combined.

4. Scoop thick batter onto prepared sheet pan in six 4 inch rounds. Or pour into six prepared mini cake pans for uniformity. Smooth batter with knife or spatula.

5. Place in oven and bake for 12 - 15 minutes, or until tops are firm to the touch and golden.
6. Remove from oven and let cool at least 5 minutes.
7. Slice in half and serve with your favorite patty or filling.

Tapioca Nut Spreads

Prep Time: 5 minutes

Cook Time: 15 minutes

Servings: 6

INGREDIENTS

1/4 cup almond flour

1/4 cup coconut flour

1/4 cup coconut milk

3 eggs

2 tablespoons unsweetened applesauce

2 tablespoons tapioca flour (or arrowroot powder)

1 teaspoon baking powder

1/2 teaspoon sea salt

INSTRUCTIONS

1. Preheat oven to 350 degrees F. Line sheet pan with parchment paper, or lightly coat with coconut oil. Or lightly coat 6 mini loaf pans with coconut oil.
2. Beat eggs, coconut milk and applesauce in medium mixing bowl with hand mixer or whisk.
3. In large mixing bowl, sift together coconut flour, almond flour, tapioca or arrowroot, baking powder and salt. Pour egg mixture into flour mixture and mix until combined.
4. Scoop thick batter onto prepared sheet pan in six long forms. Or pour into six prepared mini loaf pans for uniformity. Smooth batter with knife or spatula.

5. Place in oven and bake for 12 - 15 minutes, or until golden and tops are firm to the touch.

6. Remove from oven and let cool at least 5 minutes.

7. Slice in half or split through top, and serve with your favorite link or filling.

Tapioca Cacao Butter Meal

Prep Time: 5 minutes

Cook Time: 15 minutes

Servings: 6

INGREDIENTS

2 cups almond flour

4 eggs

1/2 cup coconut cream (or melted cacao butter)

1/2 cup arrowroot powder (or tapioca flour)

1/3 cup ground chia seed (or flax meal)

1/4 cup coconut oil

2 tablespoons unsweetened applesauce

1 teaspoon apple cider vinegar

1 teaspoon baking soda

1/2 teaspoon sea salt

INSTRUCTIONS

1. Preheat oven to 350 degrees F. Lightly coat 6 mini round cake pans with coconut oil.
2. Beat eggs, coconut oil, coconut cream, applesauce and vinegar in medium mixing bowl with hand mixer or whisk.
3. In large mixing bowl, sift together almond flour, arrowroot, chia meal, baking soda and salt. Pour egg mixture into flour mixture and mix until well combined.

4. Pour batter into prepared mini cake pans and bake for about 15 minutes, or until golden brown and toothpick inserted comes out clean.
5. Remove from oven and let cool at least 5 minutes.
6. Slice in half and serve with your favorite deli meats or sandwich salads.

NOTE: Lightly oil medium loaf pan and bake for about 25 minutes for **Sandwich Bread** loaf.

Lettuce Bacon Sandwich

Prep Time: 10 minutes*

Cook Time: 20 minutes

Servings: 2

INGREDIENTS

Sandwich Bread

8 slices nitrate-free bacon

1 large tomato

2 ribs romaine lettuce

1/2 cup arugula leaves

1/2 cup baby spinach

Honey Mustard

2 oz organic mustard

2 tablespoons sweetener*

INSTRUCTIONS

1. Preheat oven to 350 degrees F. Lightly coat 6 mini round cake pans with coconut oil. Or lightly coat loaf pan with coconut oil. Heat medium skillet over medium-high heat.

2. Prepare *Sandwich Bread* and place in oven.

3. While bread bakes, cut bacon strips in half and place in hot pan. Cook about 5 minutes, until browned and crisp on both sides. Remove skillet from heat and set bacon aside.

4. Shred romaine lettuce and toss with spinach and arugula. Thinly slice tomato. Mix mustard and sweetener in small mixing bowl.

5. Remove *Sandwich Bread* from oven and let cool about 5 minutes. Slice and spread with *Honey Mustard*.

6. Layer bottom bread slice with half lettuce mix, tomato slices and crisp bacon. Top sandwich with top bread slice and cut in half on the diagonal. Repeat with second sandwich.

7. Serve immediately.

*raw honey or agave nectar

Ground Meat Long Rolls

Prep Time: 5 minutes

Cook Time: 20 minutes

Servings: 4

INGREDIENTS

Long Roll

Meatballs

1 lb ground meat (beef, pork, chicken, turkey, bison, or any combination)

3/4 cup almond flour

1 egg

1 garlic clove

1/2 small onion

1 teaspoon dried parsley

1 teaspoon dried oregano

1/2 teaspoon ground black pepper

1/2 teaspoon sea salt

1 tablespoon coconut oil

Tomato Sauce

1 can (8 oz) organic tomato sauce

1/4 cup water

1/2 teaspoon dried oregano

1/2 teaspoon dried basil

1/2 teaspoon ground black pepper

DIRECTIONS

1. Preheat oven to 350 degrees F. Line sheet pan with parchment paper, or lightly coat with coconut oil. Or lightly coat 6 mini loaf pans with coconut oil.

2. Prepare *Long Rolls* and place in oven.

3. While bread bakes, heat large pan over medium heat and add 1 tablespoon coconut oil.

4. For *Meatballs*, peel onion and garlic and add to food processor or blender. Pulse until finely processed, but before paste forms. Or finely mince.

5. Beat egg in large bowl. Add ground meat, almond flour, spices and salt. Mix well with hands or large wooden spoon.

6. Form 24 meatballs with scoop or tablespoon, then roll in hands. Add to hot pan and brown for 10 minutes. Turn with spatula or tongs to cook on all sides.

7. Add all *Tomato Sauce* ingredients to small pot and heat over low heat. Stir and simmer, until *Meatballs* in pan are browned.

8. Add *Meatballs* to simmering *Tomato Sauce* and increase heat to medium. Simmer another 5 minutes.

9. Remove *Long Rolls* from oven and let cool about 2 minutes.

10. Slice roll along side or split through top. Use slotted spoon to fill each roll with 6 meatballs.

11. Serve hot.

Bacon Spinach Salad

Prep Time: 15 minutes

Cook Time: 15 minutes

Servings: 2

INGREDIENTS

Spinach Salad

4 cups spinach

2 eggs

8 slices nitrate-free bacon

1 avocado

1 small onion

1/4 cup almond flour

1/2 teaspoon ground black pepper

1/4 teaspoon paprika

1/4 teaspoon sea salt

Bacon Vinaigrette

Bacon drippings

2 tablespoons coconut oil

2 tablespoons apple cider vinegar

1 teaspoon sweetener*

2 teaspoons organic mustard

1/4 teaspoon ground black pepper

INSTRUCTIONS

1. Bring small pot of lightly salted water to boil. Heat medium skillet over medium-high heat.

2. Gently add eggs to boiling water with tongs and boil about 7 - 10 minutes. Then remove and rinse under cold water. Crack shells and remove whole egg. Set aside.

3. While eggs cook, chop bacon and add to hot pan. Sauté about 5 - 8 minutes, until crisp and cooked through. Remove bacon and drain on paper towel. Reserve bacon drippings. Add drippings to small bowl once cooled slightly.

4. Lightly coat hot pan with coconut oil.

5. Add almond flour and spiced to small mixing bowl. Peel onion and cut in half. Cut onion into half-moon slices. Toss with almond flour until well coated.

6. Add coated onions to hot oiled pan. Let crisp about 1 - 2 minutes, then turn and continue cooking another minute, until fully crisp. Remove onion crisps and set aside on paper towel to drain.

7. Rinse, dry and plate spinach. Slice avocado in half, pit, and slice in peel. Slice eggs.

8. Add bacon pieces, avocado slices, sliced eggs and onion crisp to salads.

9. Add *Bacon Vinaigrette* ingredients to small bowl with reserved bacon grease and whisk well. Pour over salads.

10. Serve immediately.

*stevia raw honey or agave nectar

Avocado Pickle Relish Sandwich

Prep Time: 5 minutes

Cook Time: 15 minutes

Servings: 2

INGREDIENTS

Sandwich Bread

Avocado Egg Salad

8 eggs

1 avocado

1/4 cup dill pickle relish

3 tablespoons organic mustard

2 teaspoons paprika

1/2 teaspoon ground black pepper

1/4 teaspoon sea salt

INSTRUCTIONS

1. Preheat oven to 350 degrees F. Lightly coat 6 mini round cake pans or medium loaf pan with coconut oil. Bring medium pot of lightly salted water to a boil.
2. Prepare *Sandwich Bread* and place in oven.
3. While bread bakes, gently add eggs to hot water with tongs and cook about 8 - 10 minutes.
4. Drain eggs in colander and run under cold water to cool.
5. While eggs cool, slice and pit avocado. Scoop flesh into medium mixing bowl. Add relish, mustard, salt and spices.

6. Crack eggs shells and peel. Add boiled eggs to medium mixing bowl.

7. Using a fork, mash ingredients together until smooth mixture with soft chunks forms.

8. Remove *Sandwich Bread* from oven and let cool about 5 minutes.

9. Slice bread and fill with *Avocado Egg Salad*.

10. Serve immediately. Or refrigerate about 20 minutes and serve chilled.

Broccoli Tamari Nutritional Soup

Prep Time: 10 minutes*

Servings: 2

INGREDIENTS

1 1/2 - 2 cups broccoli florets

1 red bell pepper

1 garlic clove

1/4 cup raw oil (coconut, walnut, almond, sesame, etc.)

1 cup nutritional yeast

1 tablespoon coconut aminos (or tamari)

1 tablespoon onion powder

1/2 teaspoon Celtic sea salt

1/4 teaspoon ground white pepper (or ground black pepper)

2 cups raw cashews

Water

INSTRUCTIONS

1. * Soak raw cashews in enough water to cover at least 2 hours, or overnight in refrigerator. Drain and rinse. Set aside.
2. Chop broccoli florets into pieces and set aside.
3. Seed and vein bell pepper. Peel garlic. Add to food processor or high-speed blender with soaked cashews, nutritional yeast, coconut aminos, salt, pepper and enough water to process until smooth, about 2 - 3 minutes.
4. Pour into serving bowl and top with broccoli. Serve immediately.

Sugar Free Raspberry Salad

Prep Time: 10 minutes

Servings: 1

INGREDIENTS

Salad

2 cups soft lettuce leaves (looseleaf or butterhead varieties)

1/2 cup watercress

2 tablespoons raw almonds (slivered or sliced)

1/4 cup fresh raspberries

Raspberry Vinaigrette

1/4 cup raspberries (fresh or frozen)

2 tablespoons lemon juice (or raw apple cider vinegar)

2 tablespoons raw walnuts (or raw walnut oil, coconut oil, almond oil, etc.)

1 teaspoon sweetener* (optional)

Water

INSTRUCTIONS

1. For *Salad*, rinse, dry and plate lettuce and watercress. Sprinkle almonds and fresh raspberries over greens.
2. For *Raspberry Vinaigrette*, add raspberries, lemon juice, walnuts or oil, and sweetener (optional) to food processor or high-speed blender and process until smooth, about 1 minute. Add enough water to reach desired consistency.
3. Drizzle *Raspberry Vinaigrette* over salad and serve immediately.

*stevia, raw honey or dried dates

Low Fat Oregano Caesar

Prep Time: 10 minutes

Servings: 1

INGREDIENTS

2 cups chopped romaine lettuce

Almond Parmesan

1/4 cup raw almonds

1 teaspoon raw apple cider vinegar

1 teaspoon nutritional yeast (optional)

1/4 teaspoon garlic powder

1/4 teaspoon onion powder

1/4 teaspoon dried oregano

1/4 teaspoon Celtic sea salt

Raw Caesar Dressing

2 tablespoons raw cashews (or raw sunflower seeds)

2 tablespoons raw sunflower seeds

1 tablespoon raw pine nuts (or raw sesame seeds or raw tahini)

2 tablespoons lemon juice

1 teaspoon sweetener*

1 garlic clove

3/4 teaspoon coconut aminos (or nutritional yeast)

1/2 teaspoon dried dill (optional)

Cracked or ground black pepper, to taste

Water

INSTRUCTIONS

1. Rinse, dry and plate romaine lettuce.
2. For *Almond Parmesan*, add almonds, vinegar, salt, spices and nutritional yeast (optional) to food processor or high-speed blender. Process until almonds are coarsely ground and resemble ground parmesan cheese. Set aside.
3. For *Raw Caesar Dressing*, peel garlic and add to food processor or high-speed blender with sweetener and lemon juice. Process until smooth. Then add remaining ingredients and process until smooth, about 1 - 2 minutes. Add enough water to reach desired consistency.
4. Drizzle *Raw Caesar Dressing* over salad and sprinkle with *Almond Parmesan*. Serve immediately.

* raw honey or dried dates

Lettuce Poppy Salad

Prep Time: 10 minutes*

Servings: 1

INGREDIENTS

Salad

2 cups lettuce leaves

1/2 cup dandelion leaves (optional)

2 tablespoons raw almonds (sliced or slivered)

1/4 cup fresh blueberries

Lemon Poppy Seed Dressing

3 tablespoons raw oil (coconut, walnut, almond, sesame, etc.)

2 tablespoons lemon juice

1 tablespoons sweetener*

1/4 teaspoon Celtic sea salt

1 tablespoon poppy seeds

1/4 cup raw cashews

Water

INSTRUCTIONS

1. *Soak cashews in enough water to cover for 30 minutes. Drain and rinse.
2. For *Salad*, rinse, dry and plate lettuce and dandelion leaves (optional). Sprinkle almonds and fresh blueberries over greens.

3. For *Lemon Poppy Seed Dressing*, add soaked cashews, oil, lemon juice, sweetener and salt to food processor or high-speed blender and process until smooth, about 1 - 2 minutes. Stir in poppy seeds.

4. Drizzle *Lemon Poppy Seed Dressing* over salad and serve immediately.

*stevia, raw honey or dried dates

Green Yummy Pecan Spinach Salad

Prep Time: 10 minutes

Servings: 1

INGREDIENTS

Salad

2 cups spinach leaves

1/2 cup chopped kale leaves

4 - 5 dried apricots

3 tablespoons pecans (halves or pieces)

Honey Mustard Vinaigrette

2 tablespoons raw honey (or 2 dried dates + 2 tablespoons water)

2 tablespoons ground mustard (or mustard seed)

2 tablespoons raw apple cider vinegar

3 tablespoons raw oil (coconut, walnut, almond, sesame, etc.)

3/4 teaspoons Celtic sea salt

INSTRUCTIONS

1. For *Salad*, rinse, dry and plate spinach and kale. Chop dried apricots. Sprinkle apricots and pecans over greens.

2. For *Honey Mustard Vinaigrette*, add honey, mustard, vinegar, oil and salt to food processor or high-speed blender and process until smooth, about 1 minute.

3. Drizzle *Honey Mustard Vinaigrette* over salad and serve immediately.

Veggie Lettuce Gingered Wraps

Prep Time: 35 minutes

Servings: 2

INGREDIENTS

4 large lettuce leaves (thin, flexible ribs)

1 cup cabbage (shredded)

1 small carrot

1/2 green onion

1/2 inch piece fresh ginger

1 small garlic clove

1/2 teaspoon raw sesame seeds

1/2 teaspoon coconut aminos (or tamari or raw apple cider vinegar)

1 teaspoon raw oil (sesame, coconut, walnut, almond, etc.)

Shrimp

10 - 12 medium shrimp

3/4 cup lemon juice (about 5 lemons)

1 teaspoon red pepper flakes

1/2 green onion (scallion)

Almond Sauce

2 tablespoons raw oil (sesame, coconut, walnut, almond, etc.)

1/4 cup raw almond butter (or 1/2 cup raw almonds)

1 tablespoon lemon juice (or coconut aminos or tamari)

1 tablespoons sweetener*

1/2 small mild chili pepper

Water

INSTRUCTIONS

1. For *Shrimp*, slice green onion and reserve half in small mixing bowl. Peel, devein and remove tails from shrimp. Add to separate bowl with lemon juice, remaining green onion and red pepper. Mix to combine. Shrimp should be completely covered in lemon juice. Place in refrigerator for 30 minutes, or until shrimp are opaque.

2. Peel ginger and garlic, and finely grate or mince. Add to green onion with coconut aminos and oil. Mix to combine. Set aside.

3. For *Almond Sauce*, add oil, almond butter or almonds, lemon juice, sweetener and chili pepper to food processor or high-speed blender. Process until smooth and creamy, about 1 - 2 minutes. Add enough water to reach desired consistency. Transfer to serving dish.

4. Shred cabbage and carrot and add to ginger mixture. Toss to coat.

5. Rinse, dry and plate lettuce leaves. Drain shrimp and layer onto lettuce. Top with cabbage mixture and sprinkle on sesame seeds. Roll up lettuce wraps and serve with *Almond Sauce*.

*stevia, raw honey or dried dates

Celery & Coconut Blend Salad

Prep Time: 10 minutes

Servings: 2

INGREDIENTS

2 apples

2 celery stalks

2 cups grapes

1 green onion (scallion)

1 small carrot

1 cup raw walnuts (halves or pieces)

1/3 cup raisins (or dried cranberries)

Coconut Cream Dressing

1 coconut

3/4 cup water

2 tablespoons raw walnuts

1 teaspoon mustard seeds

2 tablespoons raw apple cider vinegar (or lemon juice)

1 tablespoons sweetener*

1/2 teaspoon Celtic sea salt

INSTRUCTIONS

1. For *Coconut Cream Dressing*, remove flesh from coconut. Add 1/2 coconut and water to food processor or high-speed blender. Process until well blended and fairly smooth, about 1- 2 minutes.

2. Strain mixture through nut milk bag, cheesecloth or strainer into container. Add coconut milk back to blender with remaining coconut flesh. Process again until well blended and fairly smooth, about 1 minute.

3. Strain mixture again and place coconut cream back into blender. Reserve pulp and set aside to dry and dehydrate, then use as coconut flour.

4. Add walnuts, mustard seeds, vinegar, sweetener and salt to blender and process until smooth, about 1 - 2 minutes. Set aside.

5. Cut grapes in half and add to medium mixing bowl. Dice celery and finely grate carrot. Slice green onion. Add to medium bowl with walnuts and raisins. Seed and stem apples, then dice and add to bowl

6. Add *Coconut Cream Dressing* to bowl and mix to combine. Transfer to serving dishes and serve immediately.

7. Or refrigerate 1 hour and serve chilled.

*stevia, raw honey or dried dates

Crispy Zucchini Rolls

Prep time: 15 minutes

Cook time: 10 minutes

Serves: 2

INGREDIENTS

1 large zucchini

2-3 cloves garlic

6.5 oz artichoke hearts

½ medium onion

6 slices low sodium organic grass-fed turkey bacon

12 oz organic additive-free tomato sauce

½ green pepper

¼ tsp dried basil

¼ tsp dried oregano

¼ tsp ground black pepper

INSTRUCTIONS

1. Cut zucchini lengthwise into 8 pliable sheets. Mince the garlic and dice the onion, green pepper and artichoke.

2. Sautee bacon until it's browned. Remove the bacon from the pan and crumble. Set aside.

3. Put green pepper and onion in the pan and sautee for 2 minutes. Add garlic and sautee for another minute. Add artichoke and red sauce and bring to a bubble, about 5 minutes.

4. Add crumbled bacon and dried basil, oregano and ground black pepper to the pan. Thoroughly stir together.

For each slice of zucchini, spread cooked mixture evenly across the top and then roll up. Serve

Red Eggplant Pizza

Prep time: 10 minutes

Cook time: 8 minutes

Serves: 2

INGREDIENTS

½ large eggplant cut lengthwise

4 asparagus stalks

2 cloves garlic

1 yellow tomato

2 tsp fresh cilantro

2 tbsp extra virgin olive oil

1 cup organic red sauce

INSTRUCTIONS

1. In a medium saucepan, heat the red sauce on low and keep hot.

2. Slice the eggplant into ½ inch slices, 8 slices total. Heat 1 ½ extra virgin olive oil in a frying pan on medium heat. Cook the eggplant two minutes on one side and another two minutes on the other side. Transfer to a plate.

3. Add ½ tbsp to the pan. Slice the garlic. Rinse the asparagus and cut each asparagus stalk into 3 equal lengths.

4. Add garlic and asparagus to pan and sautee until asparagus is tender.

5. Dice yellow tomato and cilantro and mix together.

6. Place four slices of eggplant on each plate. Spoon red sauce over each slice. Cover with tomato/cilantro mixture and evenly distribute asparagus and garlic cloves.

7. Serve.

Zucchini Eggplant Dine

Prep time: 10 minutes

Cook time: 1 hour

Serves: 2

INGREDIENTS

1 large eggplant

1 medium zucchini

½ onion

1 cup mushrooms

½ green bell pepper

1 tomato

1 cup vegetable stock

2 cloves garlic

2 tbsp extra virgin olive oil

½ tsp thyme

¼ tsp parsley

INSTRUCTIONS

1. Preheat oven to 400 degrees.

2. Cut the eggplant in half lengthwise and scoop out the seeds, leaving an oblong bowl through the middle of each. Brush with 1 tbsp extra virgin olive oil. Place them cut side down on a baking sheet lined with parchment paper. Place in the oven for one hour.

3. Chop the green bell pepper, tomato, zucchini and onion. Slice the mushrooms. Combine all these ingredients in a medium saucepan with 1 tbsp extra virgin olive oil. Saute over medium heat for 4 minutes.

4. Add vegetable stock, thyme and parsley to the saucepan and let simmer until some of the liquid cooks down, approximately 10 minutes.

5. Place each half of eggplant on a plate and scoop out the vegetable mixture over the top of each.

Low Carb Chicken & Lettuce Burgers

Prep time: 15 minutes

Cook time: 8 minutes

Serves: 2

INGREDIENTS

Burger

1 eggplant

4 small organic grass-fed chicken breasts or thighs

1 tomato

1 onion

1 handful romaine lettuce

1 tbsp coconut oil

¼ tsp smoked paprika

Sauce

¼ packed cup fresh basil

2 tbsp extra virgin olive oil

1 clove garlic

2 tbsp walnuts

¼ tsp Celtic sea salt

INSTRUCTIONS

1. Combine the sauce ingredients in a food processor and puree.

2. Slice the eggplant into 8 round slices. Slice the tomato and onion into 4 slices each. Break the romaine lettuce up into smaller pieces.

3. Sprinkle the chicken with smoked paprika and combine with coconut oil in a small pan over medium heat. Sautee until cooked through and no longer pink, about 4 minutes on each side.

4. Assemble 4 burgers in the following manner: 1 slice eggplant, 1 piece chicken, 1 slice tomato, 1 slice onion, drizzled sauce, 1 slice eggplant. Secure with toothpick if desired. Serve 2 burgers to each person.

Spicy Veggie Chicken Breasts Soup

Prep time: 15 minutes

Cook time: 45 minutes

Serves: 2

INGREDIENTS

2 cups organic vegetable stock

2 organic grass-fed chicken breasts

1 red bell pepper

1 yellow bell pepper

½ onion

1 clove garlic

1 cup mango

1 tbsp extra virgin olive oil

2 tbsp lemon juice

¼ tsp Celtic sea salt

¼ tsp ground black pepper

INSTRUCTIONS

1. Cut the peppers in half. Remove the stems, cores and seeds. Line a baking sheet with aluminum foil and place the peppers in it skin

side up. Put peppers under the broiler and leave them there until the skin has begun to turn black and shriveled.

2. Remove peppers from oven, place in a plastic bag and place in refrigerator until cool.

3. Peel the skins off the peppers and throw them away. Chop the peppers.

4. Preheat oven to 350. Place chicken on a baking dish with extra virgin olive oil and lemon juice. Bake for 20 minutes or until chicken is no longer pink.

5. Chop the onion and mango and crush the garlic.

6. Place onion and garlic in a large saucepan with ½ cup vegetable stock and boil for 5 minutes. Add the rest of the stock and the roasted peppers and bring it back to a boil. Turn the heat down, cover, and let simmer for 5 minutes.

7. Using an immersion blender, blend the contents of the saucepan. Chop up the cooked chicken and place it, along with the mango, in the saucepan.

8. Season with sea salt and ground black pepper and heat through.

9. Serve.

Creamy Coconut Cocoa Fillers

Prep Time: 10 minutes

Cook Time: 20 minutes

Servings: 4

INGREDIENTS

Bun

1 cup tapioca flour/starch

1/4 - 1/3 cup coconut flour

1 egg

1/2 cup warm water

1/2 cup coconut oil

1 tablespoon sweetener*

1 teaspoon apple cider vinegar

1 tablespoon cocoa powder

1/2 teaspoon cinnamon

1/2 teaspoon baking soda

1/2 teaspoon sea salt

Filling

1 cup cashews (raw or roasted)

2 tablespoons coconut cream

2 tablespoons coconut oil

2 tablespoons cocoa powder

3 tablespoons sweetener*

1/2 teaspoon cinnamon

INSTRUCTIONS

1. Preheat oven to 350 degrees F. Line sheet pan with parchment paper or coat with coconut oil. Heat medium skillet over medium-high heat.

2. For *Filling*, add cashews, coconut oil, coconut cream, cocoa powder, sweetener and cinnamon to food processor or bullet blender and process until smooth. Add 1/2 tablespoon coconut oil at a time if needed to reach desired consistency. Set aside.

3. In medium bowl, sift together tapioca flour, 1/4 cup coconut flour, cocoa powder, cinnamon, baking soda and salt. Stir in warm water and oil.

4. Whisk egg in small mixing bowl. Add sweetenerand vinegar. Add egg mixture to flour mixture and mix until well combined.Add 1 tablespoon coconut flour or water at a time if needed to form soft and slightly sticky dough.

5. Divide dough into 4 portions and flatten into round disks. Dust your hand or rolling pin with extra tapioca flour to prevent sticking.

6. Scoop *Filling* into center of dough disks and pinch edges of dough together to create round, sealed ball.

7. Place buns sealed side down on sheet pan and pat down slightly. Bake 20 minutes, or until edges are golden brown and dough is cooked through.

8. Serve immediately. Or store in lidded container.

*stevia, raw honey or agave nectar

Spicy Ground Beef Medleys

Prep Time: 5 minutes

Cook Time: 20 minutes

Servings: 4

INGREDIENTS

16 oz (1 lb) ground meat (beef, pork, chicken, bison, or any combination)

1 cup almond flour

1 egg

1 garlic clove

1/2 small onion

1 teaspoon dried parsley

1 teaspoon dried oregano

1/2 teaspoon ground black pepper

1/2 teaspoon sea salt

Tomato Sauce

4 oz organic tomato sauce

4 oz organic crushed tomatoes

1 teaspoon dried oregano

1/2 teaspoon dried basil

1/2 teaspoon ground black pepper

DIRECTIONS

1. Preheat oven to 350 degrees. Line baking sheet with parchment or baking mat. Or prepare glass or ceramic casserole dish.

2. Pulse onion and garlic in food processor or blender until finely processed, but before paste forms. Or finely mince onion and garlic.

3. Beat egg in large bowl. Add ground meat, almond flour, spices and salt. Mix well with hands or large wooden spoon.

4. Form 18 - 24 meatballs with scoop or tablespoon, then roll in hands.

5. Arrange meatballs on lines sheet pan or in casserole dish and bake for 15 to 20 minutes, until golden brown and cooked through.

6. Add all *Tomato Sauce* ingredients to small pot and heat over medium heat. Stir and simmer about 10 minutes, until reduced and thickened.

7. Remove meatballs from oven. Toss with *Tomato Sauce* and serve hot.

8. Or allow meatballs and *Tomato Sauce* to cool, then pack in lidded containers. Serve room temperature.

Dinner Ideas

Low Fat Spicy Zucchini

Prep Time: 5 minutes

Servings: 2

INGREDIENTS

1 large zucchini

Zesty Tomato Sauce

2 medium tomatoes (or 3 plum tomatoes)

5 sundried tomatoes

2 tablespoons raw cashews (or 1 tablespoon raw cashew butter)

2 large garlic cloves

Small bunch fresh basil leaves

1 small fresh oregano sprig

Ground black pepper, to taste

Cayenne pepper, to taste

Celtic sea salt, to taste

INSTRUCTIONS

1. Carefully slice zucchini with spiralizer, vegetable peeler, or sharp knife. Sprinkle with pinch of salt, pepper and cayenne. Gently toss to coat and set aside.

2. For *Zesty Tomato Sauce*, remove basil and oregano leaves from stems. Peel garlic. Add to food processor or high-speed blender with tomatoes, sundried tomatoes, cashews or cashew butter, salt, pepper and cayenne. Process until smooth, about 1 - 2 minutes.

3. Transfer zucchini pasta to serving dishes. Top with *Zesty Tomato Sauce* and serve immediately.

Easy Zucchini Pine Nut Pesto

Prep Time: 10 minutes

Servings: 2

INGREDIENTS

1 small zucchini

1 bell pepper (or 1 carrot)

Pine Nut Pesto

2 1/2 cups fresh basil leaves

1/2 cup raw pine nuts

1 garlic clove

2 tablespoons raw oil (walnut, almond, coconut, sesame, etc.)

1/4 teaspoon ground white pepper (or ground black pepper)

1/4 teaspoon Celtic sea salt

INSTRUCTIONS

1. Carefully slice zucchini with spiralizer, vegetable peeler, or sharp knife. Carefully slice carrot with spiralizer, vegetable peeler, or grater, if using. Or remove stem, seeds and veins from bell pepper, then julienne (cut into long thin slices). Set aside.

2. For *Pine Nut Pesto*, peel garlic and add to food processor or high-speed blender with basil, 2 tablespoons pine nuts, oil, salt and pepper. Process until thick, smooth mixture forms, about 1 - 2 minutes.

3. Add *Pine Nut Pesto* to veggie pasta and toss to coat. Transfer to serving dish and top with remaining pine nuts. Serve immediately.

Zucchini Nut Parmesan Toss

Prep Time: 10 minutes

Servings: 2

INGREDIENTS

1 medium zucchini

1 carrot (or 1 small sweet potato)

Alfredo Sauce

1 cup raw cashews

1 teaspoon lemon juice (or raw apple cider vinegar)

2 garlic cloves

1/2 teaspoon dried thyme

1/2 teaspoon Celtic sea salt

Water

Walnut Parmesan

1/2 cup raw walnuts

3 tablespoons nutritional yeast

1/4 teaspoon ground white pepper (or ground black pepper)

1/2 teaspoon Celtic sea salt

INSTRUCTIONS

1. Carefully slice zucchini and carrot or sweet potato with spiralizer, vegetable peeler, or grater. Set aside.

2. For *Alfredo Sauce*, peel garlic and add to food processor or high-speed blender with cashews, lemon juice, thyme and salt. Process

until smooth mixture forms, up to 5 minutes. Add enough water to reach desired consistency. Set aside.

3. For *Walnut Parmesan*, add walnuts to clean food processor or high-speed blender and process until finely ground. Add nutritional yeast, salt and pepper. Process until coarsely ground and mixture resembling parmesan cheese forms.

4. Add *Alfredo Sauce* to veggie pasta and toss to coat. Transfer to serving dish and top with *Walnut Parmesan*. Serve immediately.

Lettuce Ribs Taco Meat

Prep Time: 35 minutes

Servings: 2

INGREDIENTS

4 large lettuce leaves (thin, flexible ribs)

1 plum tomato

1/4 red onion (or white or yellow onion)

Medium bunch cilantro

1 avocado

1/2 lime

Taco Meat

1 cup raw walnuts

1/2 cup sundried tomatoes

1/2 teaspoon ground cumin

1/4 teaspoon garlic powder

1/4 teaspoon smoked chili powder

1/4 teaspoon Celtic sea salt

Cayenne pepper, to taste

Cashew Sour Cream

1/2 cup raw cashews

1 lemon

1/8 teaspoon Celtic sea salt

3 tablespoons cup water

1/3 cup ice

INSTRUCTIONS

1. *Soak sundried tomatoes in enough water to cover at least 2 hours, or overnight in refrigerator. Drain.

2. For *Taco Meat*, add soaked tomatoes, walnuts, salt and spices to food processor or high-speed blender. Process until chunky mixture forms, about 1 minute. Set aside

3. For *Cashew Sour Cream*, add cashews, lemon juice, salt, water and ice to clean food processor or high-speed blender. Process until smooth, about 2 minutes.

4. Chop cilantro. Dice tomato. Thinly slice onion. Cut avocado in half, then remove pit and slice in peel.

5. Fill lettuce leaves with *Taco Meat*. Scoop avocado slices onto *Taco Meat*. Drizzle on *Cashew Sour Cream*. Top with diced onion and tomato, and sprinkle of chopped cilantro. Top with squeeze of lime.

6. Fold lettuce around filling and transfer to serving dish. Serve immediately.

Orange Creamy Blend

Prep Time: 5 minutes

Servings: 2

INGREDIENTS

2 cups pumpkin (chopped)

1/4 cup raw cashews (or 2 tablespoon raw cashew butter or almond butter)

1 orange

1 red bell pepper

1/2 avocado

1/4 teaspoon ground cinnamon

1/2 teaspoon ground ginger

1/2 teaspoon Celtic sea salt

1/4 cup raw pumpkin seeds

Water

INSTRUCTIONS

1. Cut avocado in half. Scoop flesh of pitted half into food processor or high-speed blender.
2. Peel and seed orange. Remove stem, seeds and veins from bell pepper. Peel and dice pumpkin. Add to processor with cashews, salt and spices. Process until smooth, up to 5 minutes. Add enough water to reach desired consistency.
3. Transfer to serving dish and top with pumpkin seeds. Serve immediately.

Spinach Shallot Salad

Prep Time: 5 minutes

Servings: 1

INGREDIENTS

Salad

2 cups spinach leaves

1/4 cup dried cranberries

2 tablespoons raw sunflower seeds

Shallot Vinaigrette

2 shallots

2 tablespoons raw sunflower seeds

2 tablespoons raw apple cider vinegar (or lemon juice)

1/2 teaspoon ground mustard (or mustard seeds)

1 1/2 tablespoons raw oil (coconut, walnut, almond, sesame, etc.)

1/4 teaspoons Celtic sea salt

INSTRUCTIONS

1. For *Salad*, rinse, dry and plate spinach. Sprinkle dried cranberries and sunflowers seeds over greens.

2. For *Shallot Vinaigrette*, peel and chop shallots. Add to food processor or high-speed blender with vinegar, sunflower seeds, mustard, oil and salt. Process until smooth, about 1 minute.

3. Drizzle *Shallot Vinaigrette* over salad and serve immediately.

Tomato Dill

Prep Time: 15 minutes*

Servings: 2

INGREDIENTS

4 medium tomatoes

1 celery stalk

1 small carrot

1 green onion (scallion)

1/3 cup sunflower seeds

1/2 red bell pepper

1/4 small red onion (or sweet onion)

1/2 teaspoon Celtic sea salt

Dill Dressing

1/2 cup raw cashews

1 tablespoon raw apple cider vinegar (or coconut aminos)

1 teaspoon ground mustard (or mustard seeds)

1/2 lemon

1 small garlic clove

2 sprigs fresh dill

1/2 teaspoon Celtic sea salt

1/4 teaspoon ground white pepper (or pinch ground black pepper)

Water

INSTRUCTIONS

1. *Soak cashews in enough water to cover at least 4 hours, or overnight in refrigerator. Drain and rinse.
2. Cut tops off tomatoes and scoop out seeds. Set aside
3. Finely dice celery and carrot. Slice green onion. Peel and dice onion. Add to medium mixing bowl. Remove stem, seeds and veins from bell pepper, then dice. Add to bowl with sprinkle of salt. Set aside.
4. For *Dill Dressing*, peel garlic and add to food processor or high-speed blender with soaked cashews, vinegar, mustard, squeeze of lemon, dill, salt and pepper. Process until smooth and creamy, about 1 - 2 minutes. Add enough water to reach desired consistency.
5. Pour *Dill Dressing* over chopped veggies. Toss to coat.
6. Plate hollowed tomatoes and stuff with *Dill Dressing* veggie mixture. Serve immediately.

Rich Mushroom Stuff

Prep Time: 35 minutes

Dehydrating Time: 1 hour

Servings: 2

INGREDIENTS

2 large Portobello mushrooms

2 tablespoons raw oil (walnut, almond, coconut, sesame, etc.)

1 tablespoon coconut aminos (or raw apple cider vinegar or tamari)

1 cup macadamia nuts

1 cup spinach

Medium bunch fresh parsley

1/3 cup sundried tomatoes

1 small lemon

1 garlic clove

1 tablespoon nutritional yeast

1 tablespoon water

1/2 teaspoon ground white pepper (or 1/4 teaspoon ground black pepper)

1/4 teaspoon Celtic sea salt

INSTRUCTIONS

1. *Soak macadamia nuts in enough water to cover at least 2 hours, or overnight in refrigerator. Soak sundried tomatoes in enough water to cover at least 4 hours, or overnight in refrigerator, if tough and chewy. Drain.

2. Cut stems off of mushrooms, if present. Chop stems and add to small mixing bowl.

3. Scrape gills from inside mushroom cap with spoon. Clean mushroom caps with damp towel. Pat dry. Add to mixing bowl with oil and coconut aminos. Toss to coat and set aside 30 - 40 minutes. Toss to coat frequently while marinating.

4. Peel garlic. Juice lemon. Add to food processor or high-speed blender with soaked tomatoes, nutritional yeast, water, salt and pepper. Process until fairly smooth, about 2 minutes.

5. Add parsley and spinach. Pulse to roughly chop greens. Mix in marinated mushroom stems, if present.

6. Line dehydrator tray with dehydrator or parchment sheet.

7. Fill mushroom caps with mixture and place on prepared dehydrator tray. Dehydrate on 105 degrees F for 1 hour.

8. Transfer to serving dish and serve immediately.

Low Fat Lettuce Gyro Meat Sandwich

Prep Time: 20 minutes*

Dehydrating Time: 15 hours

Servings: 4

INGREDIENTS

2 romaine lettuce leaves

1 large tomato

1/4 small white onion

Pita Bread

1 cup golden flax seeds

1/2 avocado

1/2 teaspoon Celtic sea salt

Water

Gyro Meat

1 1/2 cups raw walnuts

1/4 small white onion

2 garlic cloves

1 teaspoon ground cumin

1 teaspoon ground dried rosemary (or 1/2 sprig fresh rosemary)

1 teaspoon ground dried thyme

1/2 teaspoon dried oregano

1/2 teaspoon ground black pepper

1/2 teaspoon dried marjoram (optional)

1/2 teaspoon Celtic sea salt

Water

Avocado Tzatziki

1/2 small cucumber

1/2 avocado

1 teaspoon lemon juice

1/2 teaspoon apple cider vinegar (optional)

1 garlic clove

2 mint leaves

1/8 teaspoon Celtic sea salt

INSTRUCTIONS

1. *For *Pita Bread*, soak flax in 1 cup water for 6 hours.
2. Cut avocado in half. Scoop flesh of pitted half into food processor or high-speed blender. Add soaked flax and salt. Process until finely ground and well combined, about 2 minutes. Preserve remaining avocado half with pit in air tight container.
3. Prepare dehydrator trays with dehydrator or parchment sheets. Evenly spread 1/3 cup portions of batter on sheets in 1/8 inch thick circles.
4. Dehydrate at 105 degrees F for 3 hours. Flip bread over, remove sheet and continue dehydrating for 2 hours. Remove bread from the dehydrator and allow to rest for several hours to become more flexible, in zip top plastic bag if preferred.
5. *For *Gyro Meat*, soak walnuts in enough water to cover at least 4 hours, or overnight in refrigerator. Drain.

6. Peel onion and add to clean food processor or high-speed blender with soaked walnuts, salt and spices. Process until chunky mixture forms, about 1 minute.

7. Line dehydrator tray with dehydrator or parchment sheet.

8. Form mixture into loaf and flatten to 1/4 inch thick sheet. Place on lined dehydrator tray. Dehydrate on 110 degrees F for 8 - 10 hours.

9. Remove from dehydrator and slice into 1 x 6 inch strips. Set aside.

10. For *Avocado Tzatziki*, peel and mince garlic. Mince mint. Peel, seed and shred or grate cucumber. Add to small mixing bowl. Remove pit from avocado half and scoop flesh into small mixing bowl. Add lemon juice, salt and vinegar (optional). Mix well.

11. Cut tomato in half and remove seeds. Chop tomato, lettuce and onion.

12. Transfer *Pita Bread* to serving dish. Fill with *Gyro Meat* strips. Top with *Avocado Tzatziki*, and chopped tomato, lettuce and onion. Fold *Pita Bread* over filling and serve immediately.

Cheesy Macadamia Flax Meal

Prep Time: 25 minutes*

Servings: 2

INGREDIENTS

Pizza Crust

1 cup flax seeds (or 1/2 cup flax seeds + 1/2 cup chia seeds)

1 cup raw sunflower seeds

2 tablespoons raw oil (coconut, walnut, almond, sesame, etc.)

2 teaspoons dries oregano

1/4 teaspoon Celtic sea salt

Water

Pizza Sauce

1 plum tomato

2 large basil leaves

1/2 teaspoon dried oregano (or 1 teaspoon fresh oregano)

1/8 teaspoon Celtic sea salt

Macadamia Cheese

1 cup raw macadamia nuts

1/2 shallot

1 teaspoon lemon juice

1/4 teaspoon Celtic sea salt

Water

Toppings

1/2 red bell pepper

1/2 yellow bell pepper

1/4 cup grape tomatoes

1/4 white or sweet onion

Small bunch fresh basil

INSTRUCTIONS

1. *For *Macadamia Cheese*, soak nuts in enough water to cover overnight in refrigerator. Drain and rinse.

2. Peel shallot. Add to food processor or high-speed blender with soaked macadamia nuts, lemon juice, and salt. Process until smooth, up to 5 minutes. Add enough water to reach desired consistency. Set aside.

3. For *Pizza Crust*, add flax and sunflower seeds to food processor or high-speed blender. Process until finely ground. Add oregano and oil. Pulse to combine.

4. Place mixture in large mixing bowl or on parchment lined cutting board and knead in enough water to reach desired consistency. Press dough into bottom of serving dish. Set aside.

5. For *Pizza Sauce*, add tomato, basil, oregano and salt to clean food processor or high-speed blender. Process until smooth, about 1 minute. Set aside.

6. For *Toppings*, cut bell peppers in half and remove seed, stems and veins. Peel onion, Thinly slice bell pepper, onion and fresh basil. Cut grape tomatoes in half.

7. Spread *Pizza Sauce* over *Pizza Crust*. Top *Pizza Sauce* with *Macadamia Cheese*. Sprinkle with *Toppings*. Slice and serve immediately.

Spicy Zucchini Almond Crack

Prep Time: 10 minutes

Servings: 2

INGREDIENTS

1 large zucchini

1/2 teaspoon ground black pepper

Cheese Sauce

1 cup raw cashews

1/2 red bell pepper

1/3 cup nutritional yeast

1 tablespoon coconut aminos (or raw apple cider vinegar)

1/2 lemon

1/2 teaspoon smoked chili powder

1/4 teaspoonCeltic sea salt

Water

Almond Parmesan

1/2 cup raw almonds (or walnuts, cashews, etc.)

3 tablespoons nutritional yeast

1/2 teaspoon Celtic sea salt

1/2 teaspoon ground white pepper (or ground black pepper)

INSTRUCTIONS

1. *Soak cashews in enough water to cover at least 4 hours, or overnight in refrigerator. Drain and rinse.

2. Carefully slice zucchini with spiralizer, vegetable peeler, or shredding attachment on food processor. Add to medium mixing bowl with black pepper. Toss to coat and set aside.

3. Four *Cheese Sauce*, cut bell pepper in half and remove seeds, stems and veins. Add to food processor or high-speed blender with soaked cashews, nutritional yeast, coconut aminos, lemon juice, chili powder and salt. Process until smooth, about 1 - 2 minutes. Add enough water to reach desired consistency, if necessary.

4. For *Almond Parmesan*, add almonds to clean food processor or high-speed blender and process until finely ground. Add nutritional yeast, salt and pepper. Process until coarsely ground and mixture resembling parmesan cheese forms.

5. Add *Cheese Sauce* to zucchini and toss to coat. Transfer to serving dish and top with *Almond Parmesan* and crack black pepper, if preferred. Serve immediately.

Tomato Spinach Pesto

Prep Time: 15 minutes*

Servings: 4

INGREDIENTS

1 medium zucchini

Sundried Marinara

1 cup sundried tomatoes

1 plum tomato

1 dried pitted date

2 tablespoons raw oil (coconut, walnut, almond, sesame, etc.)

1 garlic clove

1/2 lemon

1/2 teaspoon dried basil

1/2 teaspoon dried oregano

1/4 teaspoon ground black pepper

Spinach Pesto

3 cups spinach

1/2 cup raw walnuts

1/4 cup raw oil (coconut, walnut, almond, sesame, etc.)

2 garlic cloves

1/2 lemon

Cashew Cheese

3/4 cup raw cashews

1 garlic clove

1 teaspoon lemon juice

1/4 Celtic sea salt

Walnut Sausage

2 cups raw walnuts

2 tablespoons coconut aminos (or tamari or raw apple cider vinegar)

1 teaspoon dried sage

1 teaspoon dried thyme

1 teaspoon fresh rosemary

1 teaspoon dried marjoram (optional)

1/2 teaspoon Celtics sea salt

INSTRUCTIONS

1. * Separately soak cashews, walnuts, and sundried tomatoes and date in enough water to cover at least 6 hours, or overnight in refrigerator. Drain and rinse nuts. Drain sundried tomatoes and date.

2. For *Sundried Marinara*, peel garlic and add to food processor or high-speed blender with soaked tomatoes and date, fresh tomato, oil, spices and squeeze of lemon. Process until finely ground and fairly smooth, about 1 - 2 minutes. Add enough water to reach desired consistency, if necessary. Set aside.

3. For *Spinach Pesto*, peel garlic and add to clean food processor or high-speed blender with soaked walnuts, spinach, oil and squeeze of lemon. Process until finely ground, about 2 minutes. Add enough water or oil to reach desired consistency, if necessary. Set aside.

4. Four *Cashew Cheese*, peel garlic and add to clean food processor or high-speed blender with soaked cashews, salt and lemon juice. Process until smooth, about 2 minutes. Add enough water to reach desired consistency, if necessary. Set aside.

5. For *Walnut Sausage*, add soaked walnuts, coconut aminos, salt and spices to clean food processor or high-speed blender. Process until coarsely ground, about 1 minute. Set aside.

6. Carefully slice zucchini into 1/8 - 1/4 inch long strips with knife or mandolin. Place layer of zucchini on serving dish. Alternate layers of *Sundried Marinara* and *Cashew Cheese*, and layers of *Spinach Pesto* and *Walnut Sausage* with zucchini layers. End with *Walnut Sausage*.

7. Slice and serve immediately. Or place inn refrigerator for 20 minute and serve chilled.

Banana with Pumpkin Soup

Prep time: 5 minutes

Cook time: approx 35 minutes

Serves: 4

INGREDIENTS

1 banana

1 onion

1 clove garlic

1 pinch nutmeg

1 ½ tbsp cinnamon

3 cups pumpkin

1 pint organic chicken stock

⅔ cup orange juice

2 tbsp extra virgin olive oil

2 tbsp sunflower seeds

¼ tsp Celtic sea salt

¼ tsp ground black pepper

INSTRUCTIONS

1. Seed, peel and cube the pumpkin.

2. Mash the banana, finely chop the onion and crush the clove of garlic. Add all three into a large saucepan with 1 tbsp extra virgin olive oil and fry gently 4-5 minutes, until soft.

3. Stir in spices and pumpkin and cook over medium heat for 6 minutes, stirring occasionally.

4. Pour in the chicken stock and orange juice. Cover and bring to a boil, then reduce heat and simmer for 20 minutes, until the pumpkin is soft.

5. Pour half the mixture into a blender or food processor and blend until smooth. Return the blended mixture to the pan and continue stirring. Add the Celtic sea salt, black pepper, cinnamon and nutmeg.

6. Add 1 tbsp extra virgin olive oil and sunflower seeds to a small pan and fry for 1-2 minutes.

Serve the soup immediately with the sunflower seeds over top, or chill 20 minutes and then serve

Kale Shallot Dish

Prep time: 10 minutes

Cook time: 15 minutes

Serves: 4

INGREDIENTS

8 cage-free eggs

2 tbsp extra virgin olive oil

1 7oz bag of Kale greens

1 shallot

¼ tsp chipotle chili pepper powder

2 cloves garlic

½ lemon

2 tbsp coconut oil

¼ tbsp ground black pepper

INSTRUCTIONS

1. Place a steamer basket in the bottom of a large pot and fill with water; if you see water rise above the bottom of the basket, pour some out. Bring the water to a boil.

2. Wash the kale and remove the stems. Mince the garlic and shallot and squeeze the juice from the lemon into a bowl.

3. In a large pan, add the eggs and extra virgin olive oil. Mixing in the chipotle chili pepper powder, scramble the eggs, breaking them up until they form many small pieces, tender yet firm.

4. Place the kale in the pot and steam until tender and bright-green.

5. Remove the kale from the pot and combine with the eggs. Add the garlic, shallot and lemon juice, drizzle the coconut oil over top and add the ground black pepper. Mix and stir thoroughly.

6. Serve immediately or chill 20 minutes and then serve.

Low Fat Chickplant Bites

Prep time: 10 minutes

Cook time: 50 minutes

Serves: 4

INGREDIENTS

4 grass-fed chicken breasts

1 eggplant

4 pinches fresh basil

¼ tsp chipotle chili pepper powder

¼ tsp curry

1 large carrot

1 red onion

1 cup coconut milk

8 wooden toothpicks

1 tbsp coconut oil

INSTRUCTIONS

1. Cut eggplant into 8 rectangles 3" long by 1" wide and 1" tall. Cut the carrot into matchsticks and dice the onion into small pieces. Cut the chicken in half lengthwise into thin filets. Soak the toothpicks in water. Preheat oven to 350.

2. Combine coconut oil, carrot, onion, 1 tsp curry, basil and chipotle chili pepper powder in a pan over medium heat. Stir together until it forms a sauce. Add eggplant and saute 7-10 minutes or until eggplant is tender.

3. Place 1 slice of eggplant on each of the chicken filets. Drizzle the contents of the pan over each of the filets; roll each fillet up around the eggplant and secure with a toothpick.

4. Place the 8 filets in the oven and bake for 35 minutes.

5. Remove from oven and pour serve 2 filets to each plate. Pour ¼ cup coconut milk and sprinkle curry over each plate's filets. Chill 20 minutes and then serve.

Spicy Roasted Pepper Chicken

Prep time: 10 minutes

Cook time: 10 minutes

Serves: 4

INGREDIENTS

4 grass-fed chicken breasts

2 tomatoes

4 olives

2 onions

¼ tsp ground black pepper

1 cup roasted red pepper

3 tbsp extra virgin olive oil

INSTRUCTIONS

1. Dice the tomatoes, chop the olives and onions, and combine them
    with ground black pepper and 2 tbsp olive oil in a bowl and mix

well into a bruschetta. Puree the roasted red pepper in a blender and set aside.

2. Combine the chicken with 1 tbsp extra virgin olive oil and cook in a pan over medium-high heat for 4 minutes, turn once, and cook another 4-6 minutes, removing from heat while still tender.

3. Place one piece of chicken on each plate and pour the roasted red pepper over each, adding bruschetta over the top. Garnish with basil and serve.

Low Carb Basil Eggplant

Prep time: 10 minutes

Cook time: 8 minutes

Serves: 4

INGREDIENTS

1 large, thick eggplant

6-8 tomatoes

4 tbsp olive oil

¼ cup fresh basil

2 cloves garlic

INSTRUCTIONS

1. Preheat the grill. Slice the eggplant lengthwise into ½" thick slices, or ensuring that you have 4 slices. Slice the tomatoes into ¼" thick slices. Combine 4 tbsp olive oil with basil and garlic in a food processor and puree together.

2. Grill the eggplant until browned, turning once, about 3-4 minutes per side.

3. Remove eggplant from the grill and lay the tomato slices out over each piece. Top with the pesto puree and serve.

Orange Zucchini Spaghetti

Prep time: 15 minutes

Cook time: 20 minutes

Serves: 4

INGREDIENTS

3 small zucchini

1 eggplant

2 green peppers

6 tomatoes

1 onion

2 medium carrots

1 four-inch sweet orange pepper

1 cup water

1 tbsp extra virgin olive oil

INSTRUCTIONS

1. Using a julienne peeler, peel zucchini, eggplant and green peppers. Green peppers may be too tough for a julienne peeler, in which case try to simulate the effect of one using a knife. Combine the above in a pan with extra virgin olive oil and saute over medium heat, stirring, for 5 minutes.

2. Meanwhile, cut tomatoes into quarters, carrots into ½" thick slices, dice sweet pepper and dice onion. In a saucepan, combine the above with water and cook over medium heat until carrot is tender, about 15 minutes. Once finished, blend using an immersion blender, or pour into a blender and puree.

3. Pour the sauce over the zucchini, eggplant and peppers and serve.

Fantasy Romaine Lettuce Salad

Prep time: 10 min

Cook time: 6-8 minutes

Serves: 4

INGREDIENTS

1 7oz bag of Romaine lettuce

1 cup strawberries

1 cup blueberries

1 cup kiwi

½ cup almonds

½ cup walnuts

2 cups coconut milk

1 tbsp arrowroot

1 tsp cinnamon

¼ tsp chipotle chili pepper powder

INSTRUCTIONS

1. Dice the fruits. In a saucepan, combine coconut milk, arrowroot, cinnamon and chipotle chili pepper powder over medium heat. Cook, stirring, for 4 minutes. Add the walnuts and almonds to the sauce and continue cooking until slightly thick.

2. Combine lettuce and fruit in a bowl and drizzle the sauce over the top. Serve immediately or chill 20 minutes and then serve.

Coconut Flour Pumpkin Roast

Prep Time: 5 minutes

Cook Time: 25 minutes

Servings: 12

INGREDIENTS

1 3/4 cups coconut flour

2 eggs

1/4 cup coconut oil

1/2 cup coconut milk

1/2 unsweetened applesauce

1/4 cup sweetener*

15oz (1 can) pumpkin puree

2 teaspoons baking soda

1 tablespoon ground cinnamon

1 teaspoon ground nutmeg

1 teaspoon sea salt

1/2 cup flaked coconut

1/4 cup pumpkin seeds

Water

INSTRUCTIONS

1. Preheat oven to 350 degrees F. Coat square baking pan with coconut oil.
2. Process eggs, coconut oil, coconut milk, applesauce and sweetener in food processor or blender until thick and lightened. Pour into medium mixing bowl. Mix in pumpkin puree and spices.

3. Mix in flour, baking soda, flaked coconut and pumpkin seeds. Stir until combined.
4. Pour batter into oiled baking pan. Bake 20 -25 minutes, or until firm but springy in center.
5. Serve warm or room temperature.

NOTE: Bake in lined or oiled muffin pan for 15 - 20 minutes for **Pumpkin Coconut Muffins**.

stevia, raw honey or agave nectar

Spicy Cocoa Bread

Prep Time: 10 minutes

Cook Time: 20 minutes

Servings: 8

INGREDIENTS

1 cup coconut flour

6 eggs

1/2 cup unsweetened applesauce

1/4 cup coconut milk

1/2 teaspoon baking soda

2 tablespoons raw cocoa powder

1/2 teaspoon ground black pepper

1/2 teaspoon salt

INSTRUCTIONS

1. Preheat oven to 350 degrees F. Coat 2 small loaf pans with coconut oil.

2. Separate eggs. In large bowl, whisk egg whites to soft peaks with hand mixer or whisk. Add yolks, applesauce and coconut milk. Mix until combined.

3. Sift in flour, baking soda, cocoa powder, black pepper and salt. Stir to combine.

4. Pour batter into oiled loaf pans. Bake 20 -25 minutes, or until firm but springy in center.

5. Serve warm or room temperature.

NOTE: Bake in largeoiled loaf pan for 30 - 40 minutes for **Cocoa Loaf.**

Low Carb Triple Flour Egg Puddings

Prep Time: 10 minutes

Cook Time:30 minutes

Servings: 12

INSTRUCTIONS

2 eggs

1/2 cup coconut milk

1/4 cup almond flour

1/4 cup arrowroot flour

1/4 cup hazelnut flour (walnut flour or cashew flour)

1 tablespoons coconut flour

1/2 teaspoon baking soda

Pinch sea salt

Coconut oil (for cooking)

INGREDIENTS

1. Preheat oven to 400 degrees F. Line muffin pan with paper liners or pour 1/2 teaspoon coconut oil into each cup and place muffin pan in oven.

2. In medium bowl, beat eggs, milk and salt. Add flours and baking soda. Mix well. Set aside for 5 minutes while batter thickens to pudding consistency.

3. Once thickened, carefully remove hot muffin pan, and use ice cream scoop or spoon to pour batter into cups. Bake 5 minutes.

4. Reduce heat to 350 degrees F and bake 20 - 25 minutes, or until puffed and golden.
5. Turn out and plate. Serve Warm.

Coconut & Almond Teasers

Prep Time: 5 minutes

Cook Time: 15 minutes

Servings: 4

INGREDIENTS

1/3 cup coconut flour

4 eggs

1/4 cup almond milk (or low-fat coconut milk)

2 tablespoons coconut oil

1 tablespoon unsweetened applesauce

1/2 teaspoon baking soda

1 teaspoon organic apple cider vinegar

Pinch sea salt

INSTRUCTIONS

1. Preheat oven to 400 degrees F. Coat 4 mini-round cake pans or 4-inch diameter oven safe ramekins with coconut oil.
2. In small mixing bowl mix baking soda and apple cider vinegar together. Set aside and allow to froth.
3. In medium bowl, beat eggs with hand mixer or whisk until thick and frothy. Add flour, milk, applesauce and salt. Combine.
4. Add baking soda and vinegar mixture and blend well until smooth and free of clumps.
5. Pour batter into pans or ramekins and bake for 12 - 15 minutes, until slightly golden and center is firm to the touch.

6. Remove muffins from oven. Loosen from sides of pan or container with knife turn out.

7. Serve warm. Muffins will have traditional **EnglishCrumpet** texture.

NOTE: For crusty, American style **English Muffins**, cut in half and toast in skillet coated with coconut oil. Press muffin down in pan with spatula and flip, browning on both sides.

stevia, raw honey or agave nectar

Yummy Chia Seed Flatbread

Prep Time: 10 minutes

Cook Time: 15 minutes

Servings: 4

INGREDIENTS

1 cup coconut flour

1/2 cup tapioca flour

1/4 cup chia seed meal (or flax meal)

2 eggs

3/4 cup water

1 teaspoon baking powder

1 teaspoon dried basil

1 teaspoon dried oregano

1/2 teaspoon ground black pepper

1/2 teaspoon sea salt

INSTRUCTIONS

1. Preheat oven to 350 degrees F. Line sheet pan with parchment paper. Prepare two additional sheets of parchment paper.
2. Whisk eggs and water in medium bowl. Set aside.
3. Combine flours, chia meal, baking powder and salt in medium bowl.
4. Pour egg mixture into flour mixture, plus spices. Mix well until dough pulls together. If dough is sticky, add 1 tablespoon of coconut flour at a time to reach proper consistency.

5. Flatten dough into basic square shape with hands on one sheet of parchment on cutting board. Cover with second sheet and use rolling pin flatten dough to about 1/8 inch thick rectangle.
6. Cut flatbread dough with pizza cutter or sharp knife into four equal pieces.
7. Gently remove top used parchment sheet and replace with fresh sheet from sheet pan. Invert sheet pan over dough and flip cutting board and sheet pan over. Replace cutting board and gently remove top used parchment sheet.
8. Use spatula to separate flatbreads. Bake in oven for 12 -15 minutes, until browned and firm. Cool and serve.

NOTE: For crisper **Flatbread**, fry flattened dough segments in oiled skillet over medium heat for about 3 minutes on each side, until puffed and browned.

Quick Asian Naan

Prep Time: 5 minutes

Cook Time: 15 minutes

Servings: 4

INGREDIENTS

1/2 cup coconut flour

4 eggs

1/4 cup coconut oil

1/2 - 2/3 cup water

1/4 tsp baking powder

1/2 teaspoons sea salt

Coconut oil (for cooking)

INSTRUCTIONS

1. Heat medium skillet over medium-high heat and coat generously with coconut oil.
2. Blend flour, eggs, oil, baking powder, salt and 1/2 cup water in a food processor or bullet blender. Process until smooth. Add liquid if batter is too thick, and coconut flour if too thin. You want a moderately thin batter.
3. Pour 1/4th of batter into hot oiled skillet. Cook until naan bubbles and browns, about 2 minutes. Then flip and cook another 2 minutes, or until golden and firm.
4. Repeat with remaining batter. Re-oil pan as necessary.
5. Drain hot naan on paper towel. Serve warm.

NOTE: For softer **Baked Naan** , bake at 425 degrees F in two (2)9-inch round cake pans generously coated with coconut oil for 10 minutes, or until cooked through.

All-Natural Baking Recipes

Weight Loss Chocó Vanilla Toss

Prep Time: 30 minutes

Cook Time: 15 minutes

Servings: 12

INGREDIENTS

Lady Fingers

1/3 cup coconut flour

3 tablespoons arrowroot powder

4 eggs

1/4 cup sweetener*

1/2 teaspoon baking powder

1/2 teaspoon vanilla

Chocolate Filling

4 oz organic dark chocolate

2 oz full-fat coconut milk

INSTRUCTIONS

1. Preheat oven to 400 degrees F. Line two sheet pans with parchment paper. Fit pastry bag with 1/2 inch round tip, or cut 1/4 inch corner off sturdy kitchen storage bag (like Ziploc®).

2. For *Lady Fingers*, beat egg yolks, sweetener and vanilla until thick and pale.

3. In separate bowl, beat egg whites to stiff peaks with hand mixer or whisk, about 8 minutes. Fold half of egg whites into egg yolk

mixture. Then sift in coconut flour, arrowroot powder and baking powder. Fold in remaining egg whites.

4. Scoop batter into pastry or storage bag. Place in tall wide contain and fold open end of bag over edge of container for easier prep.
5. Pipe 4 inch cookies onto prepared sheet pans about 2 inches apart.
6. Place in oven and bake for 8 minutes, until set and justgolden.
7. Remove cookies from oven and transfer full parchment sheet onto wire rack to cool completely. Do not try to remove warm cookies from parchment.
8. Heat 1 inch water in bottom of double boiler, or in bottom pan with metal or class bowl on top.
9. For Chocolate Filling, melt chocolate and coconut milk over double boiler until smooth.
10. Remove cooled *Lady Fingers*from parchment. Dip bottom of cookie in melted chocolate andpress against bottom of second cookie to make sandwich. Repeat with remaining cookies.
11. Serve warm. Let chocolate set for 10 minutes, in refrigerator if preferred, and serve chilled or room temperature.

*stevia, raw honey or agave nectar

Low Fat Nut Muffins

Prep Time: 5 minutes

Cook Time: 15 minutes

Servings: 4

INGREDIENTS

1/3 cup coconut flour

4 eggs

1/4 cup nut milk

2 tablespoons coconut oil

1 tablespoon unsweetened applesauce

1/2 teaspoon baking soda

1 teaspoon organic apple cider vinegar

1 teaspoon onion powder

1/4 teaspoon sea salt

1 teaspoon dehydrated onion flakes (optional)

INSTRUCTIONS

1. Preheat oven to 400 degrees F. Coat 4 mini-round cake pans or 4-inch diameter ramekins with coconut oil.

2. In small mixing bowl, mix baking soda and apple cider vinegar. Set aside and allow to froth.

3. In medium bowl, beat eggs with hand mixer or whisk until thick and lightened. Add flour, nut milk, applesauce, onion powder and salt. Mix to combine.

4. Add baking soda and vinegar mixture to medium bowl. Blend well until smooth.

5. Pour batter into prepared pans or ramekins and sprinkle on dehydrated onion flakes (optional). Bake for 12 - 15 minutes, until slightly golden and center is firm to the touch.

6. Remove muffins from oven. Loosen from sides of pans or ramekins with knife, then turn out.

7. Serve warm. Or let cool complete and serve room temperature.

Jalapeno Coconut Pretzels

Prep Time: 15 minutes

Cook Time: 20 minutes

Servings: 4

INGREDIENTS

1 cup coconut flour

1/2 cup tapioca flour

1/2 cup coconut oil

1/2 cup water

1 egg

Juice of 1/2lime

Zest if 1/2 lime

1 fresh jalapeño (or 2 oz pickled jalapeño)

2 tablespoons apple cider vinegar

1/2 teaspoon baking soda

1/2 teaspoon baking powder

1/2 teaspoon sea salt

Cilantro Lime Almond Cheese

1 cup soaked, skinless almonds*

3/4 cup water

1 tablespoons coconut oil

Juice of 1/2 lime

1 clove garlic

1/2 teaspoon sea salt

Pinch ground black pepper

Small bunch cilantro

1 1/2 cups water (for soaking)

INSTRUCTIONS

1. *Soak almonds in 1 1/2 cups water overnight. Drain and remove skins.

2. Preheat oven to 350 degrees F. Heat medium pot over medium-high heat. Line sheet pan with parchment or baking mat.

3. Add coconut oil, water, vinegar and salt to pot. Bring to a boil and remove from heat.

4. Whisk in tapioca flour. Stir with wooden spoon or soft spatula until mixture gels and comes together.

5. Stir in baking soda and baking powder. Mix for 1 minute. Mixture will foam and expand. Let mixture sit and cool about 5 minutes.

6. Remove stem, seed and veins from jalapeño and mince. Zest lime into pot, then add juice and jalapeño. Mix to incorporate.

7. Sift in coconut flour. Mix partially, then beat in egg. Blend until combined. Excess coconut flour may sit in bottom of bowl.

8. Turn out dough onto cutting board dusted with any excess coconut flour from mixture. Knead dough for 2 minutes.

9. Cut dough into 4 equal portions. Roll out pieces into ropes and twist to form classic pretzel twist. Pinch together any crumbled dough.

10. Arrange pretzels on lined sheet pan. Brush with coconut oil or full-fat coconut milk for glossy finish.

11. Place sheet pan in oven and bake about 25 minutes, until cooked through and golden.

12. For *Lime Almond Cheese*, peel garlic and add to food processor or high-speed blender with soaked almonds, coconut oil, lime juice, cilantro, salt and pepper. Process until smooth. Add water as necessary to reach desired consistency. You may process, let it rest, then process again to reach desired consistency.

13. Transfer *Cilantro Lime Almond Cheese* to serving dish.

14. Remove pretzels from oven and serve warm with *Cilantro Lime Almond Cheese*.

Low Fat Baked Bar with Creamy Topping

Prep Time: 20 minutes

Cook Time: 25 minutes

Servings: 16

INGREDIENTS

4 eggs

1/2 cup cocoa powder

1/2 cup almond flour

1/4 cup coconut oil

1/4 cup coconut milk

1/4 cup sweetener*

Juice of 1 beet

1 teaspoon vanilla

Topping

Coconut cream (settled from 1 can full-fat coconut milk)

2 - 4 tablespoons sweetener*

1/2 teaspoon vanilla

INSTRUCTIONS

1. Preheat oven to 350 degrees F. Lightly oil square baking dish or line with parchment.

2. Juice beet and add to medium mixing bowl. Add cocoa powder, eggs, coconut oil, coconut milk, sweetener and vanilla. Beat with hand mixer or whisk until well combined.

3. Pour batter into prepared baking pan and bake for 25 minutes, until set.

4. For *Topping*, beat coconut cream in medium mixing bowl until slightly thickened. Add sweetener and vanilla. Continue to beat until full thickened and fluffy, about 5 minutes.

5. Remove dish from oven and allow to cool. Frost with *Topping*.

6. Slice and serve room temperature. Or refrigerate and serve chilled.

*raw honey, agave nectar or maple syrup

Spicy Pepper Biscuits

Prep Time: 5 minutes

Cook Time: 25 minutes

Servings: 4

INGREDIENTS

3/4 cup almond flour

3/4 cup sliced almonds

3/4 cup flaked or shredded coconut

1/4 cup sweetener*

1/4 cup coconut oil

1/4 cup cocoa powder

1 teaspoon ground black pepper

1 teaspoon chili powder

1/4 teaspoon cayenne pepper

1/2 teaspoon baking soda

1 tablespoon water

INSTRUCTIONS

1. Preheat oven to 300 degrees F. Line sheet pan with parchment sheet or baking mat.

2. In medium mixing bowl, combine almond flour, sliced almonds, coconut, cocoa and spices.

3. Mix baking soda and water in small mixing bowl. Add to medium mixing bowl with sweetener and oil. Mix until combined. Add water 1 tablespoon at a time if dough is too crumbly.

4. Form 12 large biscuits and arrange on sheet pan. Flatten slightly with hand for even baking.

5. Bake for 25 - 30 minutes, until firm and browned.

6. Remove from oven and let cool about 5 minutes.

7. Serve warm. Or let cool completely and serve room temperature.

raw honey or agave nectar

Spinach Muffins

Prep Time: 10 minutes

Cook Time: 15 minutes

Servings: 12

INGREDIENTS

1 cup almond flour

2 eggs

1 cup fresh spinach

1/2 cup fresh mushrooms

1 tablespoon sweetener*

1 tablespoon apple cider vinegar

1 teaspoon baking soda

1 teaspoon baking powder

1 teaspoon ground white pepper (or black pepper)

1/2 teaspoon ground nutmeg

1/2 teaspoon dried basil

INSTRUCTIONS

1. Preheat oven to 350 degrees F. Line muffin pan with paper liners or lightly coat with coconut oil. Heat medium pan over medium-high heat.

2. Slice mushrooms and add to hot pan. Sauté about 3 minutes, then add spinach. Sauté until water evaporates, mushrooms are cooked through and spinach is wilted. Set aside.

3. Beat eggs,sweetener and vinegar in medium mixing bowl with hand mixer or whisk until thick and frothy.

4. Add sautéed veggies, almond flour, baking soda and powder and spices and mix until combined.
5. Use ice cream scoop or tablespoon to pour batter into prepared muffin pan.
6. Bake 15 - 20 minutes, until edges are golden brown and tops are firm.
7. Remove muffins from oven and let cool about 5 minutes.
8. Serve warm. Or allow to cool complete and servetemperature.

NOTE: Bake in square oiled baking pan for 30 - 35 minutes for **Spinach Mushroom Bread**.

stevia, raw honey or agave nectar

Sugar Free Almond Slice

Prep Time: 10 minutes

Cook Time: 20 minutes

Servings: 12

INGREDIENTS

2 cups almond flour

2 tablespoon sweetener*

1 egg

1 teaspoon vanilla

1/2 teaspoon baking powder

1/4 teaspoon sea salt

Filling

2 tablespoons cocoa powder

2 tablespoons sweetener*

2 teaspoons ground cinnamon

1 teaspoon ground black pepper

1/2 teaspoon vanilla

INSTRUCTIONS

1. Preheat oven to 300 degrees F. Line sheet pan with parchment or baking mat. Prepare 2 additional sheets of parchment.
2. Add flour, egg, sweetener, vanilla, baking powder and salt to medium bowl. Blend with wooden spoon, then knead with hand to form thick dough.

3. Divide dough in half. Place half of dough in small mixing bowl. Add all *Filling* ingredients to bowl and mix until well combined.

4. Roll out each half of dough separately on parchment sheets. Roll into equal rectangles.

5. Place *Filling* rectangle on top of plain dough. Use parchment to help roll dough tightly along long edge into log.

6. Use sharp knife to cut log into 1/4 round slices. Place cookies on prepared sheet pan and bake about 10 minutes, until edges are golden brown.

7. Remove from oven and let cool about 5 minutes.

8. Serve warm. Or let cool completely and serve room temperature.

*raw honey, agave nectar or maple syrup

Low Fat Tapioca Fillers

Prep Time: 10 minutes

Cook Time: 20 minutes

Servings: 8

INGREDIENTS

Dough

3 cups almond flour

3 eggs

1/2 cup dried pitted dates

1/4 cup ground chia seed (orflaxmeal)

1/4 cup tapioca flour (or arrowroot powder)

1/4 cup nut milk

2 teaspoons baking powder

1/4 teaspoon sea salt

Topping

1/2 cup dried pitted dates

1/2 cup full-fat coconut milk

Filling

2 tablespoons melted cacao butter (coconutoil)

1/2 cup dried pitted dates

2tablespoons ground cinnamon

INSTRUCTIONS

1. Preheat oven to 350 degrees F. Line muffin pan with paper liners or coat with coconut oil.Cover cutting board with parchment and coat heavily with coconut oil.

2. For *Dough*, heat nut milk in small pan over medium heat. Whisk in tapioca until combined. Remove from heat.

3. Add dates and eggs to food processor or high-speed blender. Process until thick, light mixture forms.

4. Add date mixture and tapioca mixture to medium mixing bowl. Beat in chia meal, baking soda, salt and almond flour 1 cup at a time with hand mixer or whisk.

5. Place dough onprepared parchment. Oil hands to prevent sticking and press dough into 1/2 inch thick rectangle.

6. For *Filling*, place all ingredients in clean food processor or high-speed blender and process until finely ground or smooth.

7. Roll dough intolog along edge using parchment paper. Use sharp knife or floss to slice log into rolls. Place in muffin pan.

8. For *Topping*, place dates and coconut milk in clean food processor or high-speed blender and process until smooth and creamy. Pour over rolls in muffin pan.

9. Place in oven and bake about 20 minutes, or until cinnamon bubbles and doughis firm.

10. Remove from oven and let cool at least 5 minutes.

11. Serve immediately. Or let cool completely and serve room temperature.

NOTE: Bake in oiled round baking dish or cake pan for 30 - 35 minutes for **Pan Cinnamon Rolls**.

Baked Crust Cubes

Prep Time: 25 minutes

Cook Time: 20 minutes

Servings: 12

INSTRUCTIONS

Crust

2 cups almond flour

2 eggs

2 tablespoons coconut oil

2 tablespoons cacao butter (or full-fat coconut milk)

2 tablespoons sweetener*

1 teaspoon baking powder

1/2 teaspoon baking soda

1/2 teaspoon vanilla

1/4 teaspoon ground cinnamon

1/4 teaspoon sea salt

Filling

1 cup cashews

1/4 cup dried pitted dates

1/2 cup water

2 tablespoons sweetener*

2 teaspoons ground cinnamon

1/2 teaspoon vanilla

INSTRUCTIONS

1. For *Crust*, sift almond flour into medium mixing bowl. Add baking soda and powder, vanilla, cinnamon and salt.

2. Whisk eggs and sweetener in small mixing bowl, then add to flour mixture and combine. Slowly add coconut oil and cacao butter or coconut milk until malleable dough comes together.

3. Roll in plastic wrap or wrap tightly in parchment and refrigerate for 15 minutes.

4. Preheat oven to 350 degrees F. Line sheet pan with parchment or baking mat. Cover cutting board with parchment. Heat medium pot over medium-high heat.

5. For *Filling*, bring 1/2 cup water, dates, cinnamon and vanilla to boil In small pot. Reduce heat and simmer until reduced and most liquid evaporates, about 5 minutes.

6. Add cashews to food processor or bullet blender. Process to chop cashews. Add dates and sweetener to cashews and process until dates break down and sandy mixture forms.

7. Remove dough from refrigerator. Roll dough out on parchment covered cutting board to about 1/8 inch thick rectangle with rolling pin.

8. Spread *Filling* over dough. Use sharp knife or pizza cutter to cut dough into 12 rectangles.

9. Roll up dough pieces and arrange on prepared sheet pan. Place in oven and bake 15 - 20 minutes, or until dough is golden brown and cooked through.

10. Remove from oven and allow to cool about 5 minutes.

11. Serve immediately. Or allow to cool completely and serve room temperature.

*stevia, raw honey or agave nectar

Yolk Muffins

Prep Time: 15 minutes

Cook Time: 20 minutes

Servings: 4

INGREDIENTS

3 cups almond flour

6 egg yolks (room temperature)

3 eggs (room temperature)

1/2 cup coconut oil

1/4 cup sweetener*

1 tablespoon apple cider vinegar

1 teaspoon baking soda

1/2 teaspoon sea salt

1 egg

INSTRUCTIONS

1. Preheat oven to 350 degrees F. Coat muffin pan with coconut oil or line with paper liners. Cover cutting board with parchment.

2. Add eggs and yolks to large mixing bowl. Beat with hand mixer or whisk until light and frothy. Beat in coconut oil, sweetener, vinegar, baking soda and salt. Sift in 2 1/2 cups almond flower while mixing to form sticky dough.

3. Dust parchment covered cutting board with remaining almond flour. Turn dough out onto parchment and knead for about 5 minutes.

4. Transfer dough to prepared muffin pan. Beat remaining egg in small mixing bowl and brush over bread.

5. Place in oven and bake 15 - 20 minutes, until browned and cooked through.

6. Remove from oven and let cool for 5 minutes.

7. Serve warm. Or allow to cool completely and serve room temperature.

* stevia, raw honey or agave nectar

NOTE: Bake in oiled loaf pan for 40 minutes for **Egg Bread Loaf,** or form ropes and braid dough together then bake on prepared sheet pan for 30 minutes for **Classic Egg Bread**.

Low Fat Flax Meal

Prep Time: 5 minutes

Cook Time: 25 minutes

Servings: 9

INGREDIENTS

3/4 cup almond flour

1/4 cup coconut flour

2 tablespoons flax meal (or ground chia seed)

2 eggs

1 large overripe banana

1 avocado

1/4 cup sweetener*

2 tablespoons coconut oil

1 tablespoon baking powder

1 tablespoon cinnamon

1 teaspoon ground ginger

1 teaspoon vanilla

1/2 teaspoon ground black pepper

1/2 teaspoon sea salt

1/2 cup organic banana chips (optional)

INSTRUCTIONS

1. Preheat oven to 350 degrees F. Coat square baking pan with coconut oil.

2. Slice avocado in half. Remove pit and scoop flesh into medium mixing bowl. Peel banana and add to bowl with eggs, sweetener,

and flax or chia meal. Beat with hand mixer or whisk until well blended.

3. Sift flour, baking powder, salt and spices Into banana mixture. Mix until combined. Roughly chop banana chips and fold into batter (optional).

4. Pour batter into baking pan and bake for 20 - 25 minutes, or until browned and firm in the center.

5. Remove from oven and let cool at least 5 minutes.

6. Slice and serve warm. Or allow to cool completely and serve room temperature.

NOTE: Bake in oiled loaf pan for 35 - 45 minutes for **AvocadoBanana Loaf**.

stevia, raw honey or agave nectar

Gingery Flax Meal

Prep Time: 5 minutes

Cook Time: 20 minutes

Servings: 8

INGREDIENTS

2 cups almond flour

2 tablespoons ground chia seed (or flax meal)

2 eggs

1/2 cup unsweetened applesauce

1/4 cup coconut oil

1/4 cup sweetener*

1/4 cup cocoa powder

1 tablespoon baking powder

1 teaspoon baking soda

2 tablespoons ground ginger

1 tablespoon ground cinnamon

1 teaspoon ground black pepper

1 teaspoon vanilla

1/2 teaspoon ground cloves

2 oz fresh ginger juice (optional)

INSTRUCTIONS

1. Preheat oven to 350 degrees F. Coat 2 small loaf pans with coconut oil.

2. Beat eggs in large mixing bowl with hand mixer or whisk until light and thickened, about 2 minutes. Add applesauce, oil, sweetener and ginger juice (optional). Beat well.
3. Sift all dry ingredients Into medium mixing bowl. Slowly beat flour mixture into egg mixture.
4. Pour batter into prepared loaf pans and bake for 20 - 25 minutes, or until toothpick inserted into center comes out clean.
5. Let cool at least 5 minutes. Insert knife around edges and remove brad from pan.
6. Slice and serve warm. Or let cool completely and serve room temperature.

NOTE: Bake in large oiled loaf pan for 35 - 45 minutes for **Cocoa Gingerbread Loaf**.

*raw honey, agave nectar, maple syrup, molasses

Sugar Free Cream Bread

Prep Time: 10 minutes

Cook Time: 20 minutes

Servings: 24

INGREDIENTS

2 cups coconut flour

1 cup almond flour

2 tablespoons tapioca flour (or arrowroot powder)

2 eggs

1 tart apple

1 sweet apple

1/2 cup unsweetened applesauce

1/4 cup coconut oil

1/4 cup sweetener*

1 tablespoon baking soda

1 tablespoon apple cider vinegar

1 teaspoon ground cinnamon

1 teaspoon ground ginger

1 teaspoon sea salt

1/2 teaspoon ground white pepper (or ground black pepper)

INSTRUCTIONS

1. Preheat oven to 375 degrees F. Line 2 muffin pans with paper liners or coat with coconut oil.
2. Peel, core and grate or dice apples, and place in small bowl. Pour vinegar and spices over apples. Toss to coat.

3. In medium bowl, whisk eggs with hand mixer or whisk until light and thickened, about 2 minutes. Add applesauce, sweetener and coconut oil. Blend until combined. Mix in apples.
4. Sift flours, baking soda and salt into apple mixture and mix until combined.
5. Use ice cream scoop or tablespoon to scoop equal portions of batter into muffin pans until 2/3 - 3/4 full.
6. Place in oven and bake for 15 - 20 minutes, or until golden brown and firm but springy to the touch.
7. Remove form oven and let cool at least 5 minutes.
8. Serve warm/ Or allow to cool completely and serve room temperature.

NOTE: Bake in oiled square baking pan for 35 - 45 minutes or two loaf pans for 45 - 55 minutes for **Apple Bread Loaves**.

*stevia, raw honey or agave nectar

Low Fat Blueberry Spatula

Prep Time: 10 minutes

Cook Time: 30 minutes

Servings: 12

INGREDIENTS

4 eggs

3/4 cup coconut flour

2 tablespoons arrowroot powder (or tapioca flour)

1 cup (1/2 pint) fresh blueberries

1/2 cup sweetener*

1/4 cup full-fat coconut milk

1/2 teaspoon baking powder

2 teaspoons vanilla

1 teaspoon food-grade lavender buds (ground)

1/2 teaspoon sea salt

INSTRUCTIONS

1. Preheat oven to 350 degrees F. Coat rectangular baking pan or "all-corner" specialty brownie pan with coconut oil.

2. Add blueberries to food processor or bullet blender with coconut milk and process until smooth. Set aside.

3. Beat eggs in medium mixing bowl with hand mixer or whisk. Add blueberry purée, sweetener, vanilla and lavender. Mix to combine.

4. Sift coconut flour, arrowroot or tapioca, baking powder and salt into blueberry mixture. Beat until well combined.

5. Scrape batter into prepared baking pan and smooth top with spatula.

6. Bake for 25 - 30 minutes, until center is firm and top is golden brown. Toothpick inserted into center will come out moist but mostly clean.

7. Remove from oven and allow to cool about 10 minutes.

8. Slice and serve warm. Or allow to cool completely and serve room temperature.

*stevia, raw honey or agave nectar

Chocó Muffins

Prep Time: 10 minutes

Cook Time: 25 minutes

Servings: 12

INGREDIENTS

Chocolate Coconut Cake

3/4 cup coconut flour

6 eggs

1 cup flaked or shredded coconut

1 cup unsweetened applesauce

1/2 cup coconut oil

1/2 cup coconut milk

1/2 cup sweetener*

1/2 cup dried pitted dates

1/3 cup cocoa powder

1 teaspoon vanilla

1 teaspoon baking soda

1 teaspoon baking powder

1/2 teaspoon sea salt

Chocolate Coconut Topping

Coconut cream (settled from 1 can full-fat coconut milk)

2 - 4 tablespoons sweetener*

2 tablespoons cocoa powder

1/2 teaspoon vanilla

1/2 cup flaked or shredded coconut

INSTRUCTIONS

1. Preheat oven to 325 degrees F. Line two round or square baking pans with parchment or lightly coat with coconut oil.

2. For *Chocolate Coconut Cake*, add dates, coconut milk, and half of eggs and oil to food processor or high-speed blender. Process until fairly smooth, about 1 - 2 minutes.

3. Pour date mixture into medium bowl. Add applesauce, sweetener, vanilla, and remaining eggs and oil. Beat with hand mixer or whisk until well combined.

4. Sift coconut flour, cocoa, salt, and baking soda and powder into wet ingredients. Blend until smooth. Stir in coconut.

5. Divide batter and pour into prepared baking pans and bake for about 25 minutes, or until golden and toothpick inserted into center comes out clean.

6. For *Chocolate Coconut Topping*, beat coconut cream in medium mixing bowl until slightly thickened. Add sweetener, vanilla and cocoa. Continue to beat until fully thickened and fluffy.

7. Remove cakes from oven and allow to cool. Place in refrigerator to speed cooling.

8. Frost cooled cakes and stack one on top of the other. Evenly sprinkle flaked coconut over top layer.

9. Slice and serve.

*stevia, raw honey, agave nectar or maple syrup

Almond Pecan Chocó Cookies

Prep Time: 5 minutes

Cook Time: 20 minutes

Servings: 12

INGREDIENTS

1 1/2 cups almond flour

1 1/2 cup pecans

1/4 cup cocoa powder

1/4 cup coconut oil (or melted cacao butter)

1/4 cup sweetener*

1 teaspoons vanilla

1/4 teaspoon baking soda

1/2 teaspoon sea salt

INSTRUCTIONS

1. Preheat oven to 300 degrees F. Line sheet pan with parchment or baking mat.
2. Add 1 cup pecans to food processor or high-speed blender and process until finely ground.
3. Add ground pecans to medium mixing bowl. Sift in almond flour, cocoa, baking soda and salt.
4. Chop remaining pecans and add to small mixing bowl. Add coconut oil or melted cacao butter, sweetener and vanilla to pecans. Mix to combine.
5. Pour wet mixture into dry ingredients and mix to form dough.

6. Use mini ice cream scoop or tablespoon to drop portions of dough onto prepared sheet pan.

7. Place in oven and bake 20 minutes, or until lightly browned.

8. Remove from oven and let cool at least 5 minutes.

9. Let cool completely and serve room temperature. Or serve warm.

*raw honey, agave nectar or maple syrup

Frozen Blueberry Coconut Scones

Prep Time: 5 minutes

Cook Time: 25 minutes

Servings: 8

INGREDIENTS

2 cups almond flour

1/3 cup arrowroot powder (or tapioca flour)

1 cage-free egg

1/2 cup dried or frozen blueberries

1/4 cup coconut oil

2 tablespoons sweetener*

2 teaspoons baking powder

1/2 teaspoon vanilla

1/2 teaspoon sea salt

1/4 teaspoon ground cinnamon (optional)

INSTRUCTIONS

1. Preheat oven to 350 degrees F. Line sheet pan with parchment or coat with coconut oil.

2. Whisk together almond flour, arrowroot powder, baking powder, salt, vanilla and cinnamon (optional) in medium mixing bowl.

3. In small mixing bowl, beat egg, oil and sweetener with hand mixer or whisk. Add egg mixture to dry ingredients and mix until well combined.

4. Fold in blueberries. Form dough into ball and place on sheet pan . Pat down to flatten to about 1/2 inch thick circle.

5. Cut into eight wedges with pizza cutter or sharp knife. Arrange at least 1 inch apart on sheet pan and bake for 20 - 25 minutes , or until edges are golden brown.

6. Remove from oven and let cool at least 10 minutes.

7. Serve room temperature.

raw honey, agave nectar or grade B maple syrup

Low Carb Cinnamon Bites

Prep Time: 5 minutes

Cook Time: 20 minutes

Servings: 12

INGREDIENTS

3/4 cup coconut flour

3/4 cup almond flour

1/4 cup ground chia seed (or flax meal)

2 cage-free eggs

1/2 cup raisins

1/2 cup coconut oil

1/2 cup unsweetened applesauce

1/4 cup sweetener*

2 tablespoons ground cinnamon

1 teaspoon baking powder

1 teaspoon sea salt

1/2 teaspoon ground black pepper (optional)

INSTRUCTIONS

1. Preheat oven to 350 degrees F. Line baking pan with parchment or coat with coconut oil.

2. In large bowl, whisk eggs with hand mixer or whisk until frothy and light. Add coconut oil, sweetener and applesauce. Blend until combined.

3. Sift coconut and almond flour, chia meal, baking powder, salt and spices into wet ingredients. Beat until smooth and well combined. Stir in raisins.

4. Pour batter into prepared baking pan.

5. Bake for 20 - 25 minutes, or until golden brown and firm to the touch.

6. Remove from oven and let cool about 5 minutes.

7. Slice and serve warm. Or allow to cool completely and serve room temperature.

NOTE: Bake in oiled loaf pan for 40 - 45 minutes for **Cinnamon Raison Bread** loaf.

stevia, raw honey or agave nectar

Almond Flour Chia Bagels

Prep Time:10 minutes

Cook Time: 25 minutes

Servings: 8

INGREDIENTS

2 cups almond flour

2 tablespoons coconut flour

2 tablespoons ground chia seed (or flax meal)

1 tablespoon tapioca flour (or arrowroot powder)

4 cage-free eggs

1/3 cup apple cider vinegar

2 tablespoons unsweetened applesauce

2 tablespoons sweetener*

1 teaspoon baking soda

1/2 teaspoon sea salt

INSTRUCTIONS
1. Preheat oven to 350 degrees. Lightly coat donut pan with coconut oil.
2. Add almond, coconut and tapioca flours, chia meal, baking soda and salt to food processor or bullet blender, and process for 1 minute.
3. Add eggs, sweetener, applesauce and apple cider vinegar to flour mixture and process until fully blended, about 1 - 2 minutes.
4. Carefully scoop batter into donut pan, avoiding raised middle.

5. Place in oven and bake about 20 - 25 minutes.
6. Remove and let cool about 5 minutes. Then remove from pan.
7. Slice in half and serve immediately. Or let cool completely and serve room temperature.

NOTE: Bake in 8 round mini cake pans lightly coated with coconut oil if you do not have a donut pan.

stevia, raw honey or agave nectar

Avocado Bacon Egged Muffin

Prep Time: 10 minutes

Cook Time: 15 minutes

Servings: 12

INGREDIENTS

1 cup almond flour

2 cage-free eggs

1 avocado

4 slices nitrate-free bacon

1 tablespoon sweetener*

1 teaspoon apple cider vinegar

1 teaspoon baking powder

1/4 teaspoon ground white pepper (or black pepper)

INSTRUCTIONS

1. Preheat oven to 350 degrees F. Line muffin pan with paper liners or light coat with coconut oil. Heat medium pan over medium-high heat.
2. Finely chop bacon and add to hot pan. Sauté until crisp and cooked through, about 5 minutes. Set aside.
3. Beat eggs,sweetener and vinegar in medium mixing bowl with hand mixer or whisk until thick and slightly foamy.
4. Slice avocado in half. Scoop flesh of one half into egg mixture. Add bacon and drippings, almond flour, baking powder and black pepper and mix until combined.
5. Dice remaining avocado flesh and fold into batter.

6. Use ice cream scoop or tablespoon to scoop batter into prepared muffin pan.

7. Bake about 15 - 20 minutes, until edges are golden brown and tops are firm.

8. Remove from oven and let cool for 5 minutes.

9. Serve warm. Or cool completely and serve temperature.

NOTE: Bake in square oiled baking pan for 30 - 35 minutes for **AvocadoClub Bread**.

*stevia, raw honey or agave nectar

Coconut Flour Vanilla Muffins

Prep Time: 5 minutes

Cook Time: 20 minutes

Servings: 12

INGREDIENTS

6 eggs

1/2 cup coconut flour

1/4 cup coconut oil

1/4 cup sweetener*

1 teaspoon vanilla

1 teaspoon poppy seeds

1/2 teaspoon baking soda

Juice of 2 lemons

Zest of 2 lemons

INSTRUCTIONS

1. Preheat oven to 350 degrees F. Oil muffin pan or line with paper liners.
2. Zest, *then* juice 2 lemons. Add to large mixing bowl with eggs, coconut oil, sweetener and vanilla. Beat with hand mixer or whisk until well combined.
3. Sift coconut flour and baking soda into wet ingredients, and mix until smooth. Stir in poppy seeds.
4. Use ice cream scoop or tablespoon to pour batter into prepared muffin pan.

5. Place in oven and bake for about 20 minutes, or until golden around edges and toothpick inserted into middle comes out clean.

6. Remove from oven and let cool for 5 minutes.

7. Serve warm. Or allow to cool completely and serve room temperature.

* raw honey or agave nectar

Stuffed Blackberry Almonds

Prep Time: 15 minutes

Cook Time: 20 minutes

Servings: 8

INGREDIENTS

BlackberryFilling

2 1/2 cups blackberries (fresh or frozen)

2 - 4 tablespoons sweetener*

2 tablespoons tapioca flour

1/2 teaspoon ground black pepper

Zest of 1/2 lemon

Dumplings

1/4 cup coconut flour

3/4 cup almond flour

3 tablespoons cold coconut oil

1 teaspoon baking powder

1/2 teaspoon ground cinnamon

1/4 teaspoon sea salt

2 cage-free eggs

2 tablespoon sweetener

1 teaspoon vanilla

Zest of 1/2 lemon

INSTRUCTIONS

1. For *Dumplings*, sift coconut flour, almond flour, baking powder and salt into small mixing bowl. Cut in cold coconut oil with fork until crumbly. Place in freezer for 10 minutes.

2. Preheat oven to 400 degrees F.

3. For *Blackberry Filling*, add blackberries, sweetener, black pepper and lemon zest to medium pot. Heat over medium heat and bring to simmer. Whisk in tapioca flour and simmer about 10 minutes.

4. Pour hot blackberries into casserole dish and place in hot oven.

5. In medium bowl, beat eggs, sweetener, lemon zest, cinnamon and vanilla. Add chilled flour mixture to eggs and mix until dough comes together.

6. Carefully remove dish from oven and drop 8 dumplings onto bubbling berries.

7. Return dish to oven and bake 15 - 20 min, until dumplings are golden, set and cooked through.

8. Remove dish from oven and allow to cool about 5 minutes.

9. Serve warm. Or allow to cool completely and serve room temperature.

*stevia, raw honey or agave nectar

Low Carb Vanilla Dates Bread

Prep Time: 10 minutes

Cook Time: 25 minutes

Servings: 12

INGREDIENTS

Coconut Cake

6 cage-free eggs

3/4 cup coconut flour

1 cup flaked coconut

1 cup unsweetened applesauce

1/2 cup coconut oil

1/2 cup coconut milk

1/2 cup sweetener*

1/2 cup dried pitted dates

2 teaspoons vanilla

1 teaspoon baking soda

1 teaspoon baking powder

1/2 teaspoon sea salt

Coconut Frosting

1/3 cup coconut cream (from 1 can settled full-fat coconut milk)

2 - 4 tablespoons sweetener*

1/2 teaspoon vanilla

1/2 cup flaked coconut

INSTRUCTIONS

1. Preheat oven to 325°F. Line two or square baking pans with parchment or coat lightly with coconut oil.

2. Add dates, coconut milk, and half of eggs and oil to food processor or bullet blender. Process until dates a broken down, about 1 - 2 minutes.

3. Pour date mixture into medium bowl. Add applesauce, sweetener, vanilla, and remaining eggs and oil. Beat with hand mixer or whisk until well combined.

4. Sift coconut flour, salt, and baking soda and baking powder into wet ingredients. Blend until smooth. Stir in coconut.

5. Pour batter into prepared baking pans and bake for about 25 minutes, or until golden and toothpick inserted into center comes out clean.

6. Remove from oven and allow to cool. Place in refrigerator to speed cooling.

7. For *Coconut Frosting*, beat coconut cream in medium mixing bowl until slightly thickened. Add sweetener and vanilla, and continue to beat until full thickened and fluffy.

8. Frost cooled cakes and stack one on top of the other. Evenly sprinkle flaked coconut on top layer of frosted cake.

9. Slice and serve.

*stevia, raw honey, agave nectar or maple syrup

Zucchini Egged Cake

Prep Time: 10 minutes

Cook Time: 25 minutes

Servings: 12

INGREDIENTS

1 1/2 cups almond flour

2 cage-free eggs

1 medium zucchini (1 1/2 cups grated)

1/2 cup unsweetened applesauce

1/4 cup coconut oil

1/4 - 1/2 cup sweetener*

1/4 cup cocoa powder

2 tablespoons ground chia seed (or flax meal)

1 teaspoon baking soda

1 teaspoon baking powder

1 teaspoon vanilla

1 teaspoon ground cinnamon

1 teaspoon ground black pepper

1/2 teaspoon sea salt

1/4 cup cocoa nibs or chocolate chips (optional)

INSTRUCTIONS

1. Preheat oven to 350 degrees F. Line rectangular baking pan with parchment or lightly coat with coconut oil.
2. Add eggs, coconut oil, applesauce and sweetener to food processor or bullet blender. Process until mixture is thick and lightened.

3. Grate zucchini and add to medium mixing bowl. Pour egg mixture over grated zucchini.
4. Sift almond flour, cocoa powder, chia meal, baking soda and powder, salt and spices into bowl. Beat with hand mixer or whisk to combine. Stir in cocoa nibs or chocolate chips (optional).
5. Pour batter into prepared baking pan and bake for about 25 minutes, until toothpick inserted into center comes out clean.
6. Remove from oven and let cool about 10 minutes.
7. Slice and serve warm. Or let cool completely and serve room temperature.

*stevia, raw honey or agave nectar

Spicy Cocoa Creamy Muffins

Prep Time: 10 minutes*

Cook Time: 20 minutes

Servings: 12

INGREDIENTS

1 cup almond flour

1 cup coconut flour

3 cage-free eggs

1/2 cup unsweetened applesauce

1/4 cup coconut oil

1/4 cup sweetener*

1 avocado

3 tablespoons cocoa powder

1 tablespoon baking powder

1/4 teaspoon ground black pepper

1 teaspoon sea salt

Filling

2 cups water

1 cup cashews

3 tablespoons sweetener*

2 tablespoon cocoa powder

2 - 4 tablespoons coconut milk

INSTRUCTIONS

4. *Soak cashews overnight in 2 cups water. Drain and rinse. Set aside.

5. Preheat oven to 350 degrees F. Line muffin pan with paper liners or coat with coconut oil.

6. Slice avocado in half, pit, and scoop flesh into food processor or blender. Add eggs, coconut oil, applesauce and sweetener. Process until smooth.

7. Pour avocado blend into medium mixing bowl. Sift in almond flour, cocoa powder, baking powder, salt and pepper. Beat with hand mixer or whisk until combined.

8. Pour batter into prepared muffin pan. Bake 20 -25 minutes, or until firm but springy in center.

9. For *Filling*, add soaked cashews, sweetener and cocoa powder to food processor or bullet blender. Process until smooth and creamy. Add coconut milk if necessary to reach desired consistency.

10. Remove muffins from oven and let cool.

11. Scoop out center of muffin with knife or teaspoon, and fill with *Filling*. Or transfer *Filling* to pastry bag fitted with 1/2 inch tip, insert tip into muffin and fill.

12. Serve warm or room temperature.

*stevia, raw honey or agave nectar

Comfort Food Recipes

Low Fat Zucchini Pasta

Prep Time: 20 minutes*

Servings: 2

INGREDIENTS

1 medium zucchini

1 tomato

5 sundried tomatoes

1 garlic clove

2 fresh basil leaves

1 tablespoon raw virgin coconut oil (or 2 tablespoons warm water)

1/4 teaspoon ground white pepper (or black pepper)

1/4 teaspoon sea salt

INSTRUCTIONS

1. Run zucchini through spiralizer, slice into long, thin shreds with knife, or use vegetable peeler to make flat, thin slices. Sprinkle with a pinch of salt and pepper, and gently toss to coat.

2. Add tomato, sundried tomatoes, peeled garlic, basil, coconut oil or warm water, and remaining salt and pepper to food processor or bullet blender. Process until sauce of desired consistency forms.

3. Transfer zucchini pasta to serving bowls. Top with tomato sauce and serve immediately.

4. Or refrigerate for 20 minutes and serve chilled.

Creamy Tomatoes

Prep Time: 5 minutes*

Servings: 2

INGREDIENTS

3 plum tomatoes (1 cup roughly chopped)

1 sundried tomato

1 clove garlic

2 large basil leaves

1/4 cup raw cashews

3/4 cup water

1/2 teaspoon sea salt

1/4 teaspoon ground white pepper (or ground black pepper)

INSTRUCTIONS

1. *Soak cashews for 4 hours, then drain and rinse, if preferred.

2. Add all ingredients to high-speed blender and process until smooth, about 2 minutes.

3. Pour into serving bowl and serve immediately.

Low Fat Basil Noodles

Prep Time: 10 minutes*

Servings: 2

INGREDIENTS

1 package (12 oz) kelp noodles

1/2 lemon

1 small red bell pepper

1 small carrot

Small bunch basil leaves

Crunchy Cashew Sauce

1 cup raw cashews

1 orange

1/2 lemon

1/2 teaspoon paprika

1/2 teaspoon ground oregano

1/2 teaspoon ground black pepper

1/2 teaspoon sea salt

INSTRUCTIONS

1. *Soak 3/4 cup cashews in enough water to cover at least 4 hours. Drain and rinse.
2. Rinse and drain kelp noodles. Add to medium bowl and soak 5 minutes in warm water and juice of 1/2 lemon.

3. Cut bell pepper in half, then remove stem, seeds and veins. Thinly slice bell pepper lengthwise. Use vegetable peeler or grater to make long, thin slices of carrot. Add veggies to medium mixing bowl.

4. For *Crunchy Cashew Sauce*, add soaked cashews, juice of lemon and orange, salt and spices to food processor or bullet. Process until very smooth.

5. Add drained kelp noodles to mixing bowl. Pour *Crunchy cashew Sauce* over veggies and kelp noodles. Chiffon basil leaves and chop remaining unsoaked cashews. Sprinkle over bowl.

6. Toss to coat. Transfer to serving dishes and serve immediately.

7. Or refrigerate for 20 minutes and serve chilled.

Nut Nori Dish

Prep Time: 15 minutes*

Servings: 2

INGREDIENTS

1 cup raw almonds*

1/4 cup water

2 tablespoons coconut oil

1 tablespoon lemon juice

1 tablespoon raw apple cider vinegar

1 garlic clove

1/4 teaspoon paprika

1/4 teaspoon ground black pepper

1/2 teaspoon sea salt

4 - 6 sheets dried nori (seaweed paper)

INSTRUCTIONS

1. *For *Almond Cheese*, soak almonds in enough water to cover overnight. Drain and rinse. Pop off skins and discard.

2. Add soaked almonds, water, coconut oil, lemon juice, vinegar, peeled garlic, salt and spices to food processor or bullet blender and process until smooth. Add a few extra tablespoons of water if necessary to achieve thick but smooth consistency. Transfer *Almond Cheese* to serving dish.

3. Cut noriinto small sheets and serve with *Almond Cheese*.

Sugar Free Cabbage Bowl

Prep Time: 10 minutes*

Cook Time: 20 minutes

Servings: 4

INGREDIENTS

1/2 head cabbage (2 cups shredded)

1 avocado

1 carrot

Zest of 1 lemon

Juice of 1 lemon

1 tablespoon raw honey

2 tablespoons apple cider vinegar

1 teaspoon ground white pepper (or black pepper)

1 teaspoon sea salt

INSTRUCTIONS

1. Cut avocado in half and remove pit. Scoop flesh into large mixing bowl and mash with fork.
2. Remove any tough outer leaves and core from cabbage. Shred cabbage and carrot. Add to bowl with vinegar, honey, salt and pepper. Zest *then* juice lemon, and add.
3. Toss to combine.
4. Serve immediately. Or and place in refrigerator for 20 minutes and serve chilled.

No Cook Fruit Milk

Prep Time: 5 minutes*

Cook Time: 0 minutes

Servings: 1

INGREDIENTS

1 banana

1 cup strawberries

1/2 - 1 cup water

Meat of 1/2 fresh coconut (or 1/2 cup unsweetened flaked or shredded coconut)

INSTRUCTIONS

1. *Soak flaked coconut in water for at least 4 hours.
2. Add fresh or soaked flaked coconut and water to high-speed blender. Process on high until smooth, about 1 minute.
3. Strain coconut mixture through nut milk bag or a few layers of cheese cloth. Squeeze out all excess liquid. Reserve coconut milk. Dry excess coconut, process until finely ground, and use as coconut flour.
4. Remove leaves from strawberries and chop. Peel banana.
5. Add coconut milk to blender with fruit and process on high until smooth.
6. Pour into serving glass and serve immediately.
7. Or chill in refrigerator for 20 minutes, blend for a few seconds to incorporate separated liquid, then pour into serving glass and serve chilled.

Celery with Cashew Butter

Prep Time: 5 minutes

Servings: 2

INGREDIENTS

3 celery stalks

2 tablespoons dried cranberries

Cashew Butter

1 cup cashews

1 dried pitted date

1 teaspoon raw virgin coconut oil

1/2 teaspoon ground cinnamon

1/4 teaspoon sea salt

INSTRUCTIONS

1. Add cashews, date, cinnamon, salt and coconut oil to food processor or bullet blender. Process until smooth. Let mixture rest between periods of processing to reach desired consistency, if necessary.

2. Cut celery stalks into thirds and fill wells with *Cashew Butter*. Place cranberries on cashew butter.

3. Serve room temperature. Or refrigerate 10 minutes and serve chilled.

Sugar Free Berry Bars

Prep Time: 25 minutes

Servings: 6

INGREDIENTS

1 cup dried blueberries

1/4 cup dried pitted dates

1/2 cup raw cashews

3/4 cup raw almonds

1/4 teaspoon ground cinnamon

1/4 teaspoon vanilla

Pinch sea salt

1/3 cup warm water

1 lemon

INSTRUCTIONS

1. Soak dried blueberries and dates in warm water and lemon juice for 5 - 10 minutes.
2. Add nuts to food processor or high-speed blender. Line loaf pan with parchment paper.
3. Drain fruit and add to processor with spices and pinch of lemon zest. Process for about 1 minute, until fruit and nuts break down and the mixture sticks together when pressed.
4. Scrape mixture into prepared loaf pan and press firmly into bottom with hands or spatula.
5. Place in refrigerator and chill for 10 minutes. Remove and cut into 6 bars.

6. Serve immediately. Or store in refrigerator up to 2 weeks.

Vanilla Whisk

Prep Time: 5 minutes

Servings: 2

INGREDIENTS

2 ripe peaches

1/4 cup raw honey

Pinch vanilla (optional)

Pinch cinnamon (optional)

INSTRUCTIONS

1. Add honey to small mixing bowl with optional spices. Beat with hand mixer or whisk until opaque, thick and creamy, about 5 - 10 minutes.

2. Cut peaches in half and remove pits. Slice peaches into wedges and arrange on serving dish. Transfer honey cream to serving bowl.

3. Serve immediately.

Low Fat Nuts Fudge

Prep Time: 10* minutes

Servings: 6

INGREDIENTS

1/4 cup raw cacao powder

3/4 cup raw almonds

1/2 cup raw hazelnuts (or cashews)

2 tablespoons raw virgin coconut oil

1/4 cup raw honey

1/4 cup hazelnuts (or walnuts)

INSTRUCTIONS

1. Line square baking dish with parchment paper.
2. Process almonds, 1/2 cup hazelnuts and coconut oil in food processor or bullet blender. Blend until fairly smooth and creamy.
3. Add nut butter, cocoa powder and honey to medium mixing bowl and mix well.
4. Chop remaining nuts.
5. *Spread mixture into parchment lined baking dish and top with chopped nuts. Refrigerate for 2 - 3 hours, until completely set.
6. Slice and serve chilled or room temperature.

Dried Apricot Cookies

Prep Time: 20 minutes*

Servings: 12

INGREDIENTS

3/4 cup dried apricots (1/2 cup chopped)

3/4 cup dried pitted dates (1/2 cup chopped)

1/2 cup raw macadamia nuts (frozen)

2 inch piece fresh ginger

1 teaspoon ground ginger

1/4 teaspoon ground cinnamon

1/2 cup unsweetened flakes or shredded coconut

INSTRUCTIONS

1. Place macadamia nuts in freezer for a few hours to overnight.
2. Add frozen nuts to food processor or high-speed blender. Pulse until coarsely ground.
3. Peel and finely grate fresh ginger. Add to processor with apricots, dates, ground ginger and cinnamon. Process until mixture is well broken down and sticks together.
4. Form the mixture into 12 balls and press flat. Roll cookies in coconut until well coated.
5. Cover and place in freezer for at least 10 minutes, until set up and firm.
6. Serve chilled.
7. Cover and store refrigerator or freezer until ready to serve.

Cauliflower Saffron Chops

Prep Time: 10 minutes

Cook Time: 25 minutes

Servings: 4

INGREDIENTS

1 large head cauliflower

8 oz chorizo (or other smoked sausage)

8 oz large shrimp

12 live little neck clams

12 live mussels

4 bone-in chicken thighs

1 cup chicken stock (or seafood stock)

1 small white onion

2 tablespoons smoked paprika

1 teaspoon saffron

Pinch ground black pepper

Pinch sea salt

2 tablespoons coconut oil

INSTRUCTIONS

1. Heat large pan over medium heat and add coconut oil.

2. Peel and chop onion. Add to hot oiled pan and sauté until translucent, about 2 minutes.

3. Add chicken thighs and brown about 5 minutes. Turn chicken over and cook another 5 minutes.

4. Rinse and clean clams and mussels, and remove any beards with pliers. Peel and devein shrimp. Cut chorizo into 1 inch slices. Set aside.

5. Roughly chop cauliflower and add to food processor with shredding attachment, process to "rice." Or mince cauliflower with knife.

6. Add riced or minced cauliflower to chicken and sauté 2 minutes. Add chorizo, clams, mussels and shrimp. Add paprika and saffron and sauté another 2 minutes.

7. Add chicken or seafood stock and stir to combine. Increase heat to high and bring to simmer. Reduce heat to medium-high and cover. Let simmer about 5 - 7 minutes, until liquid evaporates, shrimp is opaque, and mussels and clams open. Discard any that do not open.

8. Plate and serve hot.

Baked Ramekins

Prep Time: 10 minutes

Cook Time: 20 minutes

Servings: 2

INGREDIENTS

2 eggs

3 oz organic chocolate (semisweet or bittersweet)

2 tablespoons cocoa powder

2 tablespoons sweetener*

2 tablespoons ghee (or cacao butter)

1 teaspoon vanilla

1/4 teaspoon sea salt

1/4 teaspoon cream of tartar

1 tablespoon ghee (or cacao butter)

INSTRUCTIONS

1. Preheat oven to 375 degrees F. Grease two 8oz ceramic ramekins with 1 tablespoon ghee or cacao butter. Coat ramekins with the cocoa, and tap out excess.

2. Melt chocolate and 2 tablespoons ghee or cacao butter in large bowl over double boiler, stirring occasionally.

3. Remove chocolate mixture from heat. Add egg whites to separate medium mixing bowl, and yolks to chocolate. Whisk yolks and vanilla into chocolate until smooth. Set aside.

4. Beat egg whites, sweetener, salt and cream of tartar with hand mixer or whisk until stiff peaks form, about 8 minutes.

5. Gently fold the egg-white mixture into the chocolate mixture. Spoon batter into prepared ramekins.
6. Place in oven and bake until risen and set, about 20 minutes.
7. Remove from oven and let cool slightly. Or turn off oven and crack door open to cool slowly.
8. Serve warm.

*Stevia, agave nectar or raw honey

Sprig Muffins

Prep Time: 15 minutes

Cook Time: 25 minutes

Servings: 4

INGREDIENTS

4 cage free eggs

6 oz smoked salmon

2 sprigs fresh dill

English Muffins

1/3 cup coconut flour

1/3 cup almond flour

2 eggs

1/4 cup almond milk (or low-fat coconut milk)

2 tablespoons coconut oil

1/2 teaspoon baking soda

1 teaspoon apple cider vinegar

Hollandaise Sauce

1/2 cup ghee or coconut oil (melted)

2 egg yolks

1/2 lemon

1/4 teaspoon sea salt

INSTRUCTIONS

1. Preheat oven to 400 degrees F. Coat 2 mini-round cake pans or 4-inch diameter ceramic ramekins with coconut oil. Bring medium pot to simmer with 1 teaspoon salt and 1 teaspoon apple cider vinegar.

2. For *English Muffins*, mix baking soda and apple cider vinegar In small bowl. Set aside and allow to froth.

3. In medium mixing bowl, beat egg whites with hand mixer or whisk until thick and frothy. Add yolks, almond and coconut flour, nut milk, and coconut oil. Mix gently.

4. Add baking soda and vinegar mixture to bowl and blend well until smooth and free of clumps.

5. Pour batter into pans or ramekins and place on sheet pan. Place in oven and bake 15 -18 minutes, until golden brown and center is firm to the touch.

6. Crack eggs into 4 separate small bowls. Coat or spray metal ladle with coconut oil. Hold ladle over simmering water and pour 1 egg into coated ladle. Slowly tilt edge of ladle into hot water, filling it gently while keeping ladle just submerged in water. Do not let egg float out of ladle or submerge ladle into water entirely. Hold and cook egg about 1 - 2 minutes, until whites are opaque and yolk is warmed but still runny. Place poached egg on paper towel to drain. Repeat with remaining eggs.

7. Remove muffins from oven. Loosen from sides of cake pans or ramekins with knife and turn out onto wire rack to cool.

8. For *Hollandaise Sauce*, add egg yolks, squeeze of lemon, and salt to food processor or high-speed blender. Processor for 30

seconds. While processor or blender is running, drizzle in melted ghee or coconut oil very slowly. Process until all fat is added and emulsified and sauce thickens a bit, about 2 minutes.

9. Cut slightly cool *English Muffins* in half and transfer to serving dish.

10. Layer *English Muffin* halves with smoked salmon, then top with a poached egg. Pour *Hollandaise Sauce* over poached eggs, to taste. Sprinkle with pinch of salt and cracked black pepper, if preferred. Chop dill and sprinkle over eggs.

11. Serve immediately.

Sugar Free Creamy Chia Cakes

Prep Time: 10 minutes

Cook Time: 10 minutes

Servings: 12- 16

INGREDIENTS

1 cup coconut flour

3/4 cup cashew flour (or almond flour)

1/4 cup ground chia seed (or flax meal)

1/2 cup coconut oil

2 eggs

1/4 cup coconut crème

1/4 cup sweetener*

1/4 cup unsweetened apple sauce

1 teaspoons baking powder

1tablespoon ground cinnamon

1 teaspoon ground ginger

1 teaspoon ground white pepper (or black pepper)

1 teaspoon sea salt

2 cups fresh sliced strawberries

1/2 cup chopped walnuts (optional)

INSTRUCTIONS

1. Preheat oven to 350 degrees F. Line muffin pan with paper liners or coat with coconut oil.
2. In large bowl, whisk eggs with hand mixer or whisk until frothy and light. Add coconut oil, sweetener and applesauce.

Blend until combined. Slice strawberries, and fold in with walnuts (optional).

3. Inmedium bowl, blend flours, chia meal, baking powder, salt and spices.Stir flour blend into strawberry mixture until well combined.

4. Use ice cream scoop or tablespoon to scoop equal portions of batter into muffin pans, 1/2 - 3/4 full. Line or oil more muffin pans if excess batter remains.

5. Bake for 15 minutes, or until golden brown and firm but springy to the touch.

6. Cool enough to handle. Serve warm or room temperature.

NOTE: Bake in square oiled baking pan for 25 - 35 minutes or two oiled loaf pans for 35 - 45 minutes for **Strawberry Loaves**.

stevia, raw honey or agave nectar

Almond with Apple Sauce – A Low Carb Morning Dish

Prep Time: 10 minutes

Cook Time: 20 minutes

Servings: 24

INGREDIENTS

2 cups coconut flour

1 cup almond flour

12 ounces organic hard cider

2 eggs

1/2 cup unsweetened applesauce

1 tart apple

2 tablespoons baking powder

1 teaspoon ground nutmeg

1 teaspoon ground black pepper

1 teaspoon sea salt

INSTRUCTIONS

1. Preheat oven to 375 degrees F. Line 2 muffin pans with paper liners or coat with coconut oil.
2. Peel, core and grate or dice apple, and place in large bowl. Pour hard apple cider over apples, plus nutmeg and black pepper.

3. In medium bowl, whisk eggs with hand mixer or whisk until frothy and light. Add applesauce and blend until combined. Add egg mixture to cider and apples.
4. Slowly sift and stir flours, baking powder and salt into wet ingredients.
5. Use ice cream scoop or tablespoon to scoop equal portions of batter into muffin pans, 1/2 - 3/4 full.
6. Bake for 15 - 20 minutes, or until golden brown and firm but springy to the touch.
7. Cool enough to handle. Serve warm or room temperature.

NOTE: Bake in square oiled baking pan for 35 - 45 minutes or two oiled loaf pans for 45 - 55 minutes for **Apple Cider Loaves**.

stevia, raw honey or agave nectar

No Grain Low Carb Almond bread

Prep Time: 5 minutes

Cook Time: 20 minutes

Servings: 8

INGREDIENTS

2 cups almond flour

2 tablespoons ground chia seed (or flax meal)

2 eggs

1/2 cup unsweetened applesauce

1/4 cup coconut oil

1/4 cup sweetener*

1 tablespoon baking powder

1 teaspoon baking soda

2 tablespoons ground ginger

1 tablespoon vanilla

1 tablespoon ground cinnamon

1 teaspoon ground black pepper

1/2 teaspoon ground cloves

1/2 teaspoon cardamom (optional)

1 oz fresh ginger juice (optional)

INSTRUCTIONS

1. Preheat oven to 350 degrees F. Coat 2 small loaf pans with coconut oil.

2. In large bowl, beat eggs until light and thickened. Add applesauce, oil, sweetener and ginger juice (optional). Beat well.

3. In medium bowl, blendall dry ingredients well. Slowly stir flour mixture into egg mixture.

4. Pour batter into loaf pans and bake for 20 - 25 minutes, or until toothpick inserted into center comes out clean.

5. Let cool slightly. Insert knife around edges and remove from pan. Serve warm or room temperature.

NOTE: Bake in large oiled loaf pan for 35 - 45 minutes for **Grain-Free Gingerbread Loaf**.

raw honey, agave nectar, grade B maple syrup, molasses

Low Carb Almond Corn Muffins

Prep Time: 5 minutes

Cook Time: 15 minutes

Servings: 12

INGREDIENTS

1 cup almond flour

2 eggs

1/4 cup coconut oil

2 tablespoons unsweetened applesauce

1 teaspoon sweetener*

1 teaspoon organic apple cider vinegar

1 teaspoon baking powder

1/2 teaspoon ground turmeric (optional)

Pinch ground white pepper (optional)

INSTRUCTIONS

1. Preheat oven to 350 degrees F. Line muffin pan with paper liners or lightly coat with coconut oil.
2. Beat eggs in medium mixing bowl with hand mixer or whisk until thick and slightly frothy. Add oil, applesauce, sweetener, and vinegar and mix well.
3. Stir in almond meal, baking powder, and turmeric and white pepper (optional) until combined.
4. Use ice cream scoop or tablespoon to scoop batter into muffin pan, about 1/2 - 3/4 full.

5. Bake 15 - 18 minutes until edges are golden brown and the tops are firm.
6. Serve warm or room temperature.

NOTE: Bake in square oiled baking pan for 25 - 35 minutes for **"Corn" Bread**.

stevia, raw honey or agave nectar

Quick Delicious Almond Biscuits – Evening Snack

Prep Time: 5 minutes

Cook Time: 15 minutes

Servings: 8

INGREDIENTS

2 1/2 cups fine ground almond flour

2 eggs

1/4 cup coconut oil

1 teaspoon baking soda

1/2 teaspoon sea salt

1 tablespoon sweetener*

INSTRUCTIONS

1. Preheat oven to 350 degrees F. Line sheet pan with parchment paper.
2. Combine almond flour, baking soda and salt in medium bowl.
3. Separate egg whites into separate medium bowl, and yolk into small bowl. Beat egg whites to soft peaks with hand mixer or whisk.
4. Mix yolks, oil and sweetener into whites. Mix wet ingredients into dry to form soft, solid dough.
5. Roll dough into eight (8)1-inch thick round biscuits with hands. Place on parchment covered sheet pan and bake for 12 - 15 minutes, or until golden and firm on top. Serve warm.

NOTE: Oil square baking pan, gently press in dough, cut into 9 squares, and bake for 20 - 25 minutes for break-away pan biscuits.

*stevia, raw honey or agave nectar

Coconut & Almond Flour Fry Bread

Prep Time: 5 minutes

Cook Time: 15 minutes

Servings: 2

INGREDIENTS

1 cup coconut flour

1 cup almond flour (or cashew flour)

1/4 cup tapioca flour/starch

3 eggs

1/2 cup coconut oil

1/2 cup full-fat coconut milk

1 teaspoon baking powder

2 tablespoons sweetener*

Pinch sea salt

Water (for thinning)

Coconut oil (for cooking)

INSTRUCTIONS

1. Heat medium skillet over medium-high heat and coat generously with coconut oil.
2. Blend eggs, oil, milk and sweetener in food processor or bullet blender until smooth and a bit airy.
3. In medium bowl, combine flours, baking powder and salt. Add egg mixture and combine to form soft dough. If too tough, add water 1 tablespoon at a time.

4. Form dough into 2 large flat rounds with hands. Place 1 round in pan and cook about 3 minutes, or until puffed and browned. Flip fry bread with tongs or spatula and cook another 3 minutes, or until golden and cooked through.
5. Repeat with remaining dough. Re-oil pan as necessary.
6. Drain hot fry bread on paper towel. Serve warm.

NOTE: For **BakedFry Bread** , generously coat two 9-inch round cake pans with coconut oil. Press dough into pans and brush tops with coconut oil. Bake at 425 degrees F in for 15 minutes, or until cooked through and golden.

stevia, raw honey or agave nectar

Crunchy Coconut Crackers

Prep Time: 10 minutes

Cook Time: 10 minutes

Servings: 4

INGREDIENTS

1 cup coconut flour

3/4 cup almond flour

4 egg whites

1/4 cup coconut oil

1/4 cup coconut crème

1/4 cup sweetener

1/2 cup flaked coconut

1 teaspoon vanilla

1/2 teaspoon baking soda

3/4 teaspoon sea salt

1/2 teaspoon ground white pepper (or black pepper)

INSTRUCTIONS

1. Preheat oven to 375 degrees F. Line sheet pan with parchment paper or coat with coconut oil. Prepare two additional sheets of parchment.

2. Whisk egg and oil with hand mixer or whisk until blended and slightly frothy. Add sweetener, coconut crème and vanilla, and continue blending.

3. Sift in half of flour, baking soda, vanilla, salt and pepper. Add coconut flakes. Sift in remaining flour. Stir and bring dough together.

4. Form dough into rectangle and flatten with hands on parchment. Cover with second sheet of parchment and flatten to about 1/4 inch with rolling pin. Remove top layer of parchment.

5. Cut rectangles from dough with pizza cutter or sharp knife. Carefully flip dough onto sheet pan. Arrange at least 1/2 inch apart on sheet pan.

6. Bake for about 10 minutes, or until crisp and golden brown. Remove and let cool. Serve room temperature.

Chocó Dip with Celery

Prep Time: 10 minutes*

Servings: 2

INGREDIENTS

2 - 3 medium celery stalks

Hazelnut Spread

1 cup raw hazelnuts

1/4 cup raw cocoa powder

1/4 cup raw honey (or dried pitted dates)

1/2 teaspoon vanilla

Pinch Celtic sea salt

Raw nut milk (optional)

Water

INSTRUCTIONS

1. *Soak hazelnuts in enough water to cover overnight in refrigerator. Drain and rinse. Soak dates in enough water to cover overnight in refrigerator, if using. Drain.

2. Add soaked hazelnuts to food processor or high-speed blender and process until smooth, up to 10 minutes. Scrape down sides as needed.

3. Add honey or soaked dates, cocoa powder, vanilla and salt to processor. Process until smooth, about 1 minute. Add nut milk to reach desired consistency (optional).

7. Cut celery stalks into 3 in pieces. Scoop *Hazelnut Spread* into wells of celery with small spoon or knife. Fill wells completely and smooth with knife or back of spoon. Transfer filled celery to serving dish.

8. Serve immediately. Or refrigerate 20 minutes and serve chilled.

Chocó Pecan Snack

Prep Time: 10 minutes*

Servings: 6

INGREDIENTS

1 cup raw pecans

1 cup dried pitted dates

2 tablespoons raw coconut butter (or cacao butter)

1/4 cup raw cocoa powder

1/4 cup shredded or flaked coconut

1/4 teaspoon Celtic sea salt

INSTRUCTIONS

1. Line square baking dish with parchment paper. Allow coconut or cacao butter to soften.

2. Add pecans to food processor or high-speed blender and process until finely ground, about 1 minute.

3. Add dates and coconut or cacao butter and process until mixture sticks together, about 1 - 2 minutes.

4. Add cocoa, coconut and salt. Process until well ground but not completely smooth.

5. *Transfer mixture to parchment lined baking dish and firmly press into bottom with hands or spatula. Refrigerate until set, about 2 hours.

6. Remove from refrigerator. Slice and serve chilled. Or allow to warm to room temperature and serve.

Vanilla Chocó Chip Cookies

Prep Time: 35 minutes

Servings: 6

INGREDIENTS

1 1/4 cups fine almond flour

3 teaspoons coconut flour

1/3 cup dried pitted dates

1/4 cup raw coconut butter (or cacao butter)

1 teaspoon vanilla

1/8 teaspoon Celtic sea salt

1/2 cup raw chocolate chips (or chopped raw chocolate bark or cacao nibs)

INSTRUCTIONS

1. Allow coconut or cacao butter to soften at room temperature. Line sheet pan with parchment paper.
2. Add softened butter and dates to food processor or high speed blender. Process until fairly smooth, about 2 minutes.
3. Add half of almond and coconut flours, and process for about 1 minute. Add remaining flour, vanilla and salt. Process until mixture comes together. Stir in chocolate or cacao nibs.
4. Use tablespoon or mini ice cream scoop to form dough into balls. Set on lined sheet pan and place in refrigerator 30 minutes.
5. Remove from refrigerator and serve chilled. Or allow to warm slightly and serve room temperature.

Sugar-Free Coconut Ice Cream

Prep Time: 30 minutes*

Servings: 4

INGREDIENTS

2 1/2 cups shredded or flaked coconut (or 3 mature coconuts + 1/2 cups shredded or flaked coconut)

3/4 cup dried pitted dates (or raw honey)

1 1/2 teaspoons vanilla

Water

INSTRUCTIONS

1. *Freeze ice cream maker canister for at least 12 hours.
2. *Soak 2 cups coconut in 4 cups water at least 6 hours, or overnight in refrigerator. Soak dates in enough water to cover at least 6 hours, or overnight in refrigerator (if using). Drain.
3. Add soaked coconut, soaking liquid and dates (if using) to food processor or high-speed blender.
4. Or remove flesh from fresh coconuts and add to high-speed blender with 4 cups water and dates (if using). Process until well blended and fairly smooth, about 1 - 2 minutes.
5. Strain mixture through nut milk bag, cheesecloth or strainer back into blender. Reserve pulp and set aside to dry and dehydrate, then use as coconut flour.
6. Add 1/2 cup shredded or flaked coconut, vanilla and honey (if using) to coconut milk. Process to combine, about 10 seconds.

7. Assemble ice cream maker and turn on. Slowly pour mixture into running ice cream maker. Let machine run for about 20 minutes, until ice cream is set.

8. Transfer to serving dish and serve immediately.

On the Go Recipes

Low Fat Apricot Pine Bars

Prep Time: 25 minutes

Servings: 6

INGREDIENTS

1 cup raw cashews

2 lemons

1/2 cup dried pineapple

1/2 cup flaked or shredded coconut

1/4 cup dried apricots

1/4 teaspoon ground ginger

1/4 teaspoon vanilla

Pinch Celtic sea salt

1/3 cup warm water

INSTRUCTIONS

1. Zest *then* juice lemons into small mixing bowl. Reserve half of juice and zest.
2. Soak dried pineapple and apricots in warm water and juice and zest of 1 lemon for 5 - 10 minutes.
3. Line loaf pan with parchment paper.
4. Add cashews to food processor or high-speed blender. Drain fruit and add to processor with coconut, salt, spices, and lemon juice and zest. Process for about 1 minute, until fruit and nuts break down and mixture sticks together when pressed.
5. Transfer mixture to prepared loaf pan and press firmly into bottom with hands or spatula.

6. Place in refrigerator and chill for 10 minutes. Remove and cut into 6 bars.

7. Serve immediately. Or store refrigerated in airtight container up to 2 weeks.

Sugar Free Gingerly Almond Crackers

Prep Time: 5 minutes

Dehydrating Time: 4 - 8 hours

Servings: 12

INGREDIENTS

2 cups raw almond flour

1 1/2 cups dried pitted dates

4 inch piece fresh ginger

2 tablespoons raw coconut oil (or raw cacao or coconut butter)

2 tablespoons raw honey

2 teaspoons ground ginger

1 teaspoons ground cinnamon

1/2 teaspoon ground black pepper (or ground white pepper)

1/2 teaspoon vanilla

1/4 teaspoon Celtic sea salt

INSTRUCTIONS

1. Peel and grate ginger. Add to food processor or high-speed blender with almond flour, dates, oil or butter, honey, salt and spices . Process until mixture is well ground and comes together, about 2 minutes.
2. Line dehydrator trays with dehydrator or parchment sheets.
3. Form mixture into 12 - 24 balls and place on lined dehydrator trays. Press to flatten.
4. Place in dehydrator and dehydrate at 115 degrees F for 4 - 8 hours, until desired crispiness is reached.

5. Remove from dehydrator and transfer to serving dish. Serve immediately. Or store in airtight container.

Dates Almond Wafers

Prep Time: 10 minutes*

Dehydrating Time: 8 - 16 hours

Servings: 12

INGREDIENTS

1/2 cup almonds

3/4 cups cashews

1/3 cup dates

1/4 cup raw cocoa powder

1 tablespoon raw oil (coconut, walnut, almond, sesame, etc.)

1 teaspoon vanilla

1/4 teaspoon Celtic sea salt

Water

INSTRUCTIONS

1. *Soak almonds in enough water to cover for at least 6 hours, or overnight in refrigerator. Drain and rinse. Soak cashews and dates in enough water to cover for at least 1 hour. Drain.

2. Add soaked almonds and cashews to food processor or high-speed blender. Process until finely ground, about 1 - 2 minutes.

3. Add dates, cocoa, oil, vanilla and salt to processor. Process until mixture is well combined and sticks together, about 1 - 2 minutes.

4. Line dehydrator trays with dehydrator or parchment sheets.

5. Form mixture into 12 balls and place on dehydrator or parchment sheets. Press to flatten.

6. Place in dehydrator and dehydrate at 115 degrees F for about 8 - 16 hours, depending on desired crispiness.
7. Remove from dehydrator and transfer to serving dish. Serve immediately. Or store in airtight container.

Very Berry Biscuits

Prep Time: 5 minutes

Servings: 4

INGREDIENTS

1/2 cup raw almonds

1/2 cup raw pumpkin seeds

1/2 cup cashews

1/4 cup golden raisins

1/4 cup dried blueberries

1/4 cup dried strawberries

INSTRUCTIONS

1. Roughly chop dried strawberries. Add to medium mixing bowl with fruit and nuts. Mix to combine.

2. Transfer to serving dish and serve immediately. Or store in airtight container.

Dried Apricot Packers

Prep Time: 10 minutes

Servings: 4

INGREDIENTS

1 cup dried apricots

1/4 cup raw cashews

2 - 3 tablespoons dried cranberries

2 - 3 tablespoons dried blueberries

INSTRUCTIONS

1. Roughly chop cashews and add too small mixing bowl with cranberries and blueberries. Mix to combine.

2. Open apricots slightly to reveal pocket. Take pinch of mixed nuts and fruit and stuff apricots. Leave a little room to pinch apricot closed.

3. Transfer to serving dish and serve immediately. Cr store in airtight container.

Sugar Free Creamy Dates Energy Bars

Prep Time: 35 minutes

Servings: 6

INGREDIENTS

1 cup dried pitted dates

1 cup flaked or shredded coconut

3/4 cup golden flax seed

1/2 cup raw sunflower seeds (or raw pine nuts)

1/4 cup cacao butter (or coconut butter)

1/4 teaspoon Celtic sea salt

1 teaspoon vanilla

1/4cup cacao nibs (or raw chocolate chunks) (optional)

INSTRUCTIONS

1. Line baking dish with parchment paper. Allow cacao butter or coconut butter to soften.
2. Add flax to food processor or high-speed blender and process until finely ground, about 2 minutes. Add sunflower seeds and cacao butter. Process until fairly smooth, about 2 minutes.
3. Add dates, coconut, vanilla and salt. Process until mixture comes together, about 1 minute.
4. Transfer to medium mixing bowl and stir in cacao nibs or raw chocolate chunks (optional).
5. Transfer mixture to lined dish and press into bottom with hands or spatula. Place in freezer at least 25 minutes.

6. Remove from freezer. Slice and serve chilled. Or allow to warm slightly and serve.

Rich Fruit & Flax Slice

Prep Time: 10 minutes

Dehydrating Time: 6 - 8 hours

Servings: 8

INGREDIENTS

1 apple

1 lemon

1 orange

1 cup dried pitted dates

1/2 cup dried apricots

1/3 cup ground flax seed

1/2 cup raw pecans

1/2 cup raw walnuts

1 teaspoon ground cinnamon

1 teaspoon ground ginger

1/4 teaspoon Celtic sea salt

INSTRUCTIONS

1. Add pecans, walnuts and flax to food processor or high-speed blender. Process until finely ground, about 1 minute.

2. Peel and roughly chop apple around core. Zest *then* juice orange and lemon. Add to food processor or high-speed blender with dates, apricots, cinnamon, ginger and salt. Process until mixture is well ground and sticks together, about 2 minutes.

3. Line dehydrator tray with dehydrator or parchment sheet.

4. Form mixture into 2 loaves and place on lined dehydrator tray. Place in dehydrator and dehydrate at 115 degrees F for 2 hours. Reduce to 110 degrees F and continue to dehydrate for another 4 - 6 hours.

5. Remove from dehydrator and slice. Transfer to serving dish and serve immediately. Or store in airtight container.

Low Fat Cashew Balls

Prep Time: 5 minutes

Dehydrating Time: 8 - 12 hours

Servings: 12

INGREDIENTS

1 cup cashews

1 cup flaked or shredded coconut

1 lemon

1 tablespoon raw honey

INSTRUCTIONS

1. Add cashews to food processor or high-speed blender and process until finely ground, about 1 minute.
2. Zest *then* juice lemon. Add to processor with coconut and honey. Process until mixture is well combined and sticks together, about 1 - 2 minutes.
3. Line dehydrator trays with dehydrator or parchment sheets.
4. Form mixture into 12 - 24 balls and place on dehydrator or parchment sheets. Press to flatten.
5. Place in dehydrator and dehydrate on 115 degrees F for about 8 - 12 hours, until desired crispiness is reached.
6. Remove from dehydrator and transfer to serving dish. Serve immediately. Or store in airtight container.

Whole Flax Orange Crackers

Prep Time: 10 minutes

Dehydrating Time: 12 - 20 hours

Servings: 4

INGREDIENTS

2 cups ground flax seed

2/3 cup whole flax seed

1 1/3 cups raw sunflower seeds

1/2 cup raw black sesame seeds (or white sesame seeds)

1 orange

1 teaspoon ground cinnamon

1 teaspoon ground ginger

1 teaspoon ground black pepper (or ground white pepper)

1 teaspoon Celtic sea salt

2 2/3 cups water

INSTRUCTIONS

1. Place parchment paper or dehydrator sheets on dehydrator trays.
2. Zest *then* juice orange and add to large mixing bowl with water, seeds, salt and spices. Mix until well combined.
3. Spread batter on lined dehydrator trays. Place trays in dehydrator and set to 120 degrees F for 1 hour. Reduce temperature to 105 degrees F for 12 - 20.
4. After 4 hours, remove trays from dehydrator and use knife to score crackers in preferred shape and size. Place back in dehydrator and continue dehydrating.

5. Remove trays from dehydrator. Peel crackers from sheets and break apart along score lines. Place crackers directly on dehydrator tray and continue dehydrating another 6 - 12 hours, depending on desired crispness.

6. Remove crackers from dehydrator and serve immediately. Or store in an airtight container.

Kale Almond Bites

Prep Time: 10 minutes

Cook Time: 12 - 24 hours

Servings: 8

INGREDIENTS

2 cups raw almonds

1 kale head (about 3 cups chopped)

1 cup raw coconut flour

1 cup golden flax seed

1 cup water

3/4 cup nutritional yeast

1/2 teaspoon ground black pepper

1 teaspoon smoked paprika

1 teaspoon Celtic sea salt

INSTRUCTIONS

1. Place parchment paper or dehydrator sheets on dehydrator trays.
2. Add flax to food processor or high-speed blender and process until finely ground, about 2 minutes. Transfer to small mixing bowl with water. Mix to combine and set aside.
3. Add almonds to food processor or high-speed blender and process until finely ground, about 2 minutes. Transfer to medium mixing bowl.
4. Wash and spin dry kale. Add to processor and pulse to finely chop, about 1 minute. Add to mixing bowl with nutritional yeast, salt and spices. Add soaked flax and mix until dough forms.

5. Transfer dough to lined dehydrator trays and press into 1/4 inch thick rectangle with hands or rolling pin. Score with knife or pizza cutter into desired shapes.

6. Place tray in dehydrator and dehydrate at 120 degrees F for 2 hours. Reduce temperature to 115 degrees F and continue to dehydrate for 8 - 12 hours.

7. After 6 hours, remove trays from dehydrator and flip crackers. Place back in dehydrator and continue dehydrating .

Remove crackers from dehydrator and serve immediately. Or store in airtight container

Triple Berry Flax Bars

Prep Time: 30 minutes

Servings: 8

INGREDIENTS

1 cup raw cashews (or 3/4 cup raw cashew butter)

2 tablespoons flax seed (or chia seed)

1/2 cup dried pitted dates

1/2 cup shredded or flaked coconut

1/3 cup raw pumpkin seeds

1/3 cup raw walnuts

1/3 cup raw almonds

1/4 cup dried cherries

1/4 cup dried blueberries

1/4cup dried raspberries

1/2 teaspoon ground ginger (optional)

1/2 teaspoon vanilla

1 teaspoon Celtic sea salt

INSTRUCTIONS

1. Line loaf pan with parchment paper.
2. Add flax or chia to food processor or high-speed blender and process until finely ground, about 1 - 2 minutes.
3. Add cashews (if using)and process until thick, smooth paste forms, up to 5 minutes.
4. Add dates and process until thick, fairly smooth mixture forms about 1 - 2 minutes. Transfer to medium mixing bowl.

5. Add coconut, pumpkin seeds, walnuts, almonds, vanilla, salt, dried fruit and ginger (optional). Add prepared cashew butter (if using). Stir to combine with large wooden spoon.

6. Transfer mixture to parchment lined pan and firmly press into bottom with hands or spatula. Place in refrigerator for 20 minutes.

7. Remove from refrigerator and cut into bars. Serve chilled. Or allow to warm to room temperature and serve.

Fruit Strips

Prep Time: 5 minutes

Dehydrating Time: 6 hours

Servings: 6

INGREDIENTS

1 ripe banana

2 cups fresh strawberries (chopped)

2 tablespoons ground chia or flax seed (optional)

Water (optional)

INSTRUCTIONS

1. Remove stems from fresh strawberries and roughly chop. Peel and chop banana. Add to food processor or high-speed blender and process until smooth, about 1 minute.

2. Add ground chia or flax to processor and process with enough water to reach desired consistency. Mixture should be spreadable but not runny.

3. Line dehydrator tray with dehydrator or parchment sheet.

4. Spread mixture on sheet 1/4 inch thick in large rectangle with spatula. Place in dehydrator and dehydrate at 115 degrees F for 4 hours.

5. Remove from dehydrator and use offset spatula to gently peel leather from sheet and flip over. Place back in dehydrator directly on tray and continue to dehydrate for 2 hours.

6. Remove from dehydrator and cut into strips. Or roll up and cut into logs. Transfer to serving dish and serve immediately.

Carrot Toss Crisp

Prep Time: 5 minutes

Dehydrating Time: 18 - 24 hours

Servings: 4

INGREDIENTS

2 large carrots

1 tablespoon raw oil (coconut, walnut, almond, sesame, etc.) (optional)

1/2 teaspoon Celtic sea salt (optional)

INSTRUCTIONS

1. Carefully cut carrot into 1/16 - 1/8 inch thick slices with sharp knife, mandolin or food processor with slicing attachment.
2. Add sliced carrot to medium mixing bowl with oil and salt and toss to coat (optional).
3. Add single layer of sliced carrots to dehydrator tray and place in dehydrator. Dehydrate at 115 degrees F for 12 hours.
4. Remove dehydrator trays and turn over carrot slices. Place trays back in dehydrator and continue dehydrating for 6 - 12 hours, depending on desired crispiness.
5. Remove carrots from dehydrator and transfer to serving dish. Serve immediately. Or store in airtight container.

Mango Mouth Bites

Prep Time: 10 minutes

Dehydrating Time: 24 hours

Servings: 4

INGREDIENTS

2 ripe mangos

INSTRUCTIONS

1. Cut mango around pit, and cut into 1/4 inch thick slices. Then remove peel. Or slice then peel.
2. Add single layer of sliced mango to dehydrator trays. Place in dehydrator and dehydrate at 115 degrees F for 24 hours, or until dried but not crisp.
3. Remove mango from dehydrator and transfer to serving dish. Serve immediately. Or store in airtight container.

Pineapple Slices

Prep Time: 10 minutes

Dehydrating Time: 12 - 16 hours

Servings: 4

INGREDIENTS

1 ripe pineapple

INSTRUCTIONS

1. Peel pineapple and cut around core into 1/4 - 1/3 inch thick slices.
2. Add single layer of sliced pineapple to dehydrator trays. Place in dehydrator and dehydrate at 115 degrees F for 12 - 16 hours, or until dried but not crisp.
3. Remove pineapple from dehydrator and transfer to serving dish. Serve immediately. Or store in airtight container.

Sugar – Free Crunchy Banana

Prep Time: 5 minutes

Dehydrating Time: 12 - 16 hours

Servings: 4

INGREDIENTS

4 ripe or overripe bananas

INSTRUCTIONS

1. Peel bananas and cut into 1/4 - 1/3 inch thick slices lengthwise or crosswise.
2. Line dehydrator trays with dehydrator or parchment sheet. Add single layer of sliced banana to lined dehydrator trays .
3. Place bananas in dehydrator and dehydrate on 115 degrees F for 12 - 16 hours, depending on desired crispiness.
4. Remove bananas from dehydrator and transfer to serving dish. Serve immediately. Or store in airtight container.

Low Carb Apple Chips

Prep Time: 5 minutes

Dehydrating Time: 10 - 14 hours

Servings: 4

INGREDIENTS

4 sweet apples

1 teaspoon ground cinnamon (optional)

INSTRUCTIONS

1. Carefully cut apple around core into 1/16 - 1/8 inch thick slices with sharp knife, mandolin or food processor with slicing attachment.

2. Add single layer of sliced apple to dehydrator tray . Sprinkle with cinnamon (optional). Place in dehydrator and dehydrate at 105 degrees F for 10 - 14 hours, depending on desired crispiness.

3. Remove apples from dehydrator and transfer to serving dish. Serve immediately. Or store in airtight container.

Cauliflower Popcorns

Prep Time: 5 minutes

Dehydrating Time: 12 - 24 hours

Servings: 2

INGREDIENTS

2 cups cauliflower florets (roughly chopped)

1 teaspoon raw oil (coconut, walnuts, almond, sesame, etc.)

1 teaspoon coconut aminos (or tamari, apple cider vinegar or lemon juice)

3 tablespoons nutritional yeast

1 teaspoon Celtic sea salt

INSTRUCTIONS

1. Cut larger cauliflower florets into smaller pieces. Add to medium mixing bowl or container with well-fitting lid.
2. Evenly sprinkle on oil, coconut aminos, nutritional yeast and salt.
3. Secure lid on bowl or container and shake well until cauliflower is evenly coated.
4. Line dehydrator trays with dehydrator or parchment sheets.
5. Add single layer of coated cauliflower to lined dehydrator trays and place in dehydrator. Dehydrate at 115 degrees F for 12 - 24 hours, until desired crispiness is reached. Turn cauliflower over half way through dehydrating.
6. Remove from dehydrator and transfer to serving dish. Serve immediately.

Spicy Chicken Tubes

Prep time: 5 minutes

Cook time: 3 minutes

INGREDIENTS

4 slices of chicken deli meat

1 tbsp olive oil

1 small onion

1 red bell pepper

1 avocado

¼ tsp garlic powder

INSTRUCTIONS

1. Remove the nut from the avocado and mash it into a paste. Chop the pepper and onion into small pieces.

2. Combine the garlic powder, pepper and onion in the bowl with the avocado and mix well.

3. Add the olive oil in a pan over low heat and heat the chicken mildly, turning frequently, for 3 minutes.

4. Remove the chicken from heat and place ¼ of the avocado/pepper/onion mixture onto each piece.

5. Wrap the chicken up into tubes and serve.

Butter Pancakes

Prep time: 5 minutes

Cook time: 2-4 minutes

INGREDIENTS

½ cup organic cashew butter

½ cup organic applesauce

2 cage-free eggs

¼ tsp cinnamon

INSTRUCTIONS

1. Mix cashew butter, applesauce, cinnamon and eggs in a bowl.

2. Pour dollops of this mixture into a frying pan over medium heat. Flip as you would a pancake and cook until thickened, about 1 to 2 minutes on each side. Continue until all the mixture is gone.

3. Serve.

Flour Free Egg Toasts

Prep time: 15 minutes

Cook time: 40 minutes

INGREDIENTS

¾ cup cashew butter

6 cage-free eggs

2 tbsp raw, unfiltered honey

¼ cup coconut oil

½ tsp apple cider vinegar

¼ cup ground golden flax

3 tbsp coconut flour

1 tsp baking soda

½ tsp Celtic sea salt

INSTRUCTIONS

1. Preheat oven to 350 degrees. Line an 8x4 pan with parchment paper and use enough coconut oil to coat the bottom.

2. Use an immersion blender to blend the cashew butter, eggs, honey, remaining coconut oil and apple cider vinegar together. Set aside.

3. Combine the flax, coconut flour, baking soda and Celtic sea salt together.

4. Combine the two mixes by mixing the dry into the wet. Pour into the greased and lined loaf pan and bake for 40 minutes.

5. Remove from oven and cool for 10 minutes before removing from pan.

6. Slice the bread to desired thickness and toast.

Spicy Pesto Turkey Wrap

Prep time: 20 minutes

Serves: 2

INGREDIENTS

Wrap

6 slices organic grass-fed deli turkey

½ red bell pepper

6 cherry tomatoes

½ avocado

6 arugula leaves

Pesto

½ packed cup fresh basil

2 tbsp extra virgin olive oil

2 tbsp almonds

1 clove garlic

¼ tsp Celtic sea salt

INSTRUCTIONS

1. Chop the red bell pepper. Mash the avocado.

2. Combine the pesto ingredients in a food processor and puree. Set aside.

3. Stack 3 slices of turkey and spread half the pesto across the top. Across the middle, lay ¼ cup chopped red bell pepper, half the avocado mash, 3 cherry tomatoes and 3 arugula leaves. Repeat this process for the other 3 slices of turkey and wrap them both up, securing with toothpicks. Serve.

Spicy Seafood Wraps

Prep time: 15 minutes

Serves: 2

INGREDIENTS

4 sheets of Nori

1 can of tuna fish

1 tbsp extra virgin olive oil

1 tsp dried mustard

2 scallions

¼ cup raspberry

1 tbsp raw unfiltered honey

INSTRUCTIONS

1. Moisten the Nori to make it pliable. Chop the scallions.

2. Combine the tuna, extra virgin olive oil, dried mustard and chopped scallions and mix them together into a blend.

3. Spread the blend into each piece of Nori and wrap them up. Drizzle with honey and place raspberries on top. Serve.

Spicy Celery & Chicken Wraps

Prep time: 15 minutes

Serves: 2

INGREDIENTS

6 slices organic grass-fed deli chicken

1 jalapeno

2 stalks celery

½ avocado

1 tbsp fresh basil

INSTRUCTIONS

1. Chop the jalapeno pepper and mash the avocado. Slice the celery into stalks that fit the diameter of a slice of deli chicken meat.

2. Stack 3 slices of deli chicken and spread the avocado mash across the middle. Place the celery through the center, sprinkle the basil across the middle and then evenly distribute the jalapeno slices. Wrap the chicken up and secure with toothpicks. Save enough of each ingredient to repeat this process across the other 3 slices of deli chicken. Serve.

Green Spicy Chicken Salad

Prep time: 15 minutes

Cook time: 10 minutes

Serves: 2

INGREDIENTS

2 cups spinach leaves

10 shrimp

1 organic grass-fed chicken breast

½ cup soaked wakame

½ cup cherry tomatoes

½ yellow bell pepper

1 carrot

raspberry vinaigrette for dressing

1 tbsp extra virgin olive oil

¼ tsp Celtic sea salt

¼ tsp smoked paprika

INSTRUCTIONS

1. Chop the chicken breast into slices. Peel and devein the shrimp.

    Chop the yellow bell pepper. Using a vegetable grater, shred the carrot. Sprinkle the smoked paprika and Celtic sea salt over the chicken slices.

2. Using a small pot and steamer rack, steam the shrimp until they are opaque and have curled into a C-shape.

3. In a small pan, cook the chicken in 1 tbsp extra virgin olive oil over medium heat for 4 minutes, turn and cook another 4 minutes until no longer pink.

4. In each bowl, add the spinach and wakame first as a base. Then add the other ingredients and drizzle raspberry vinaigrette as dressing. Serve.

Quick Snacks

Raw Nut Snack

Prep Time: 10 minutes

Servings: 2

INGREDIENTS

2 apples

Almond Butter

1 cup raw almonds

1 teaspoon raw oil (almond, coconut, walnut, etc.) (optional)

1 teaspoon raw honey

1/4 teaspoon Celtic sea salt

Pinch ground cinnamon

INSTRUCTIONS

1. Add almonds to food processor or high-speed blender. Process until smooth, up to 10 minutes. Scrape down sides as needed. Add oil to reach desired consistency (optional).
2. Add honey, salt and cinnamon and process to incorporate, about 30 seconds.
3. Remove core, seeds and stems from apples. Leave apples hollow in center.
4. Scoop *Almond Butter* into hollowed apples with small spoon or knife. Fill hollows completely and transfer stuffed apples to serving dish.
5. Serve immediately. Or refrigerate 20 minutes and serve chilled.

Creamy Cinnamon Snacks

Prep Time: 5 minutes*

Servings: 2

INGREDIENTS

2 large carrots

Cashew Cream

1 cup raw cashews

4 dried pitted dates

1/2 teaspoon ground cinnamon

1/4 teaspoon Celtic sea salt

Pinch ground ginger

Water (or raw nut milk)

INSTRUCTIONS

1. *Soak cashews in enough water to cover at least 6 hours, or overnight in refrigerator. Drain and rinse. Soak dates in enough water to cover at least 6 hours, or overnight in refrigerator. Drain.

2. Add cashews, dates, cinnamon, salt and ginger to food processor or high-speed blender. Process until smooth, about 2 minutes. Add enough water or raw nut milk to reach desired consistency. Transfer to serving dish.

3. Cut carrots into sticks and transfer to serving dish.

4. Serve carrots with Cashew Cream immediately. Or refrigerate 20 minutes and serve chilled.

Apples with Lemon Juice

Prep Time: 5 minutes

Servings: 2

INGREDIENTS

2 large apples

1 tablespoon lemon juice (or apple cider vinegar)

1/2 teaspoon vanilla (optional)

1/2 teaspoon cinnamon (optional)

INSTRUCTIONS

1. Peel apples, if preferred. Remove core, seeds and stem, then roughly chop. Add to food processor or high-speed blender with lemon juice, vanilla and cinnamon (optional). Process until smooth, about 1 - 2 minutes. Scrape down as necessary.
2. Transfer to serving dish and serve immediately. Or refrigerate for 20 minutes and serve chilled.

Energy Reviving Cookies

Prep Time: 30 minutes

Servings: 8

INGREDIENTS

1 cup raw cashews (or 3/4 cup raw cashew butter)

2 tablespoons flax seed (or chia seed)

1/2 cup dried pitted dates

1/2 cup shredded or flaked coconut

1/3 cup raw pumpkin seeds

1/3 cup raw walnuts

1/3 cup raw almonds

1/4 cup raw chocolate chips (or cacao nibs)

1/4 cup dried goji or noni berries (optional)

1/2 teaspoon ground cinnamon

1/2 teaspoon vanilla

1 teaspoon Celtic sea salt

INSTRUCTIONS

1. Line loaf pan with parchment paper.
2. Add flax or chia to food processor or high-speed blender and process until finely ground, about 1 - 2 minutes.
3. Add cashews (if using)and process until thick, smooth paste forms, up to 5 minutes.
4. Add dates and process until thick, fairly smooth mixture forms about 1 - 2 minutes. Transfer to medium mixing bowl.

5. Add coconut, pumpkin seeds, walnuts, almonds, cinnamon, vanilla, salt, chocolate chips or cacao nibs, and goji or noni berries (optional). Add prepared cashew butter (if using). Stir to combine with large wooden spoon.

6. Transfer mixture to parchment lined pan and firmly press into bottom with hands or spatula. Place in refrigerator for 20 minutes.

7. Remove from refrigerator and cut into bars. Serve chilled. Or allow to warm to room temperature and serve.

Strawberry Logs

Prep Time: 15 minutes

Dehydrating Time: 6 hours

Servings: 6

INGREDIENTS

1 cup dried strawberries

2 cups fresh strawberries

2 tablespoons ground chia or flax seed (optional)

Water (optional)

INSTRUCTIONS

1. Remove stems from fresh strawberries and roughly chop. Add to food processor or high-speed blender and process until smooth, about 30 seconds.

2. Add dried strawberries and process until smooth, about 1 minute. Set aside 10 minutes.

3. Add ground chia or flax to processor and process with enough water to reach desired consistency. Mixture should be spreadable but not runny.

4. Line dehydrator tray with dehydrator or parchment sheet.

5. Spread mixture on sheet 1/4 inch thick in large rectangle with spatula. Place in dehydrator and dehydrate on 115 degrees F for 4 hours.

6. Remove from dehydrator and use offset spatula to gently peel leather from sheet and flip over. Place back in dehydrator and continue to dehydrate for 2 hours.

7. Remove from dehydrator and cut into strips. Or roll up and cut into logs. Transfer to serving dish and serve immediately.

Weight Loss Tangerine Sticks

Prep Time: 10 minutes*

Servings: 12

INGREDIENTS

2 cups orange or tangerine juice (about 9 oranges or 15 tangerines)

1/2 cup shredded or flaked coconut (or 1 mature coconut)

Water

Ice pop maker, toothpicks or popsicle sticks

INSTRUCTIONS

1. *Freeze ice pop maker or ice cube tray for at least 30 minutes.
2. *Soak flaked coconut in 2/3 - 3/4 cups water at least 6 hours, or overnight in refrigerator.
3. Add soaked coconut and soaking liquid to food processor or high-speed blender.
4. Or remove flesh from fresh coconut and add to high-speed blender with 2/3 - 3/4 cups water. Process until well blended and fairly smooth, about 1 - 2 minutes.
5. Strain mixture through nut milk bag, cheesecloth or strainer back into blender. Reserve pulp and set aside to dry and dehydrate, then use as coconut flour.
6. Juice oranges and add to blender. Process until well combined, about 30 seconds.
7. Remove ice pop maker or ice cube tray from freezer. Pour mixture into wells and fill 3/4 full. Place in freezer about 20 minutes.

8. Place ice pop maker sticks, toothpicks or popsicle sticks into well. Return to freezer about 20 minutes.

9. Remove ice pops from freezer and serve immediately.

Creamy Spicy Onion Bites

Prep Time: 15 minutes*

Dehydrating Time: 16 - 24 hours

Servings: 4

INGREDIENTS

Almond Milk/Coating

1/2 cup raw almonds

Water

Onions Rings

2 cups *Almond Milk*

1/3 cup *Almond Coating*

1 medium onion (sweet or white)

1/4 cup ground flax seed (or 1/3 cup whole flax seeds)

1 teaspoon smoked paprika

1/4 teaspoon ground white pepper (or pinch ground black pepper)

1/4 teaspoon Celtic sea salt

INSTRUCTIONS

1. *For *Almond Milk/Coating*, soak almonds in enough water to cover at least 6 hours, or overnight in refrigerator. Drain and pop off skins, if preferred.
2. Add soaked almonds to high-speed blender with 2 cups water. Process until well blended and almost smooth, about 1- 2 minutes.
3. Strain mixture through nut milk bag, cheesecloth or strainer into medium lidded container. Reserve almond pulp.

4. For *Almond Coating* Line dehydrator tray with dehydrator or parchment sheets. Spread almond pulp on lined dehydrator tray and dehydrate into on 110 degrees F for 6 - 12 hours, until completely dry.

5. Peel and slice onion. Add to *Almond Milk* and gently mix to coat. Let onions soak while *Almond Coating* dehydrates.

6. Remove *Almond Coating* from dehydrator and set aside. Line dehydrator trays with dehydrator or parchment sheets.

7. Add flax to food processor or high-speed blender with 1/3 cup *Almond Coating*, salt and spices. Process until finely ground. Split into 2 batches and transfer to shallow dishes.

8. Drain onions, reserving *Almond Milk*. Dip onions into *Almond Milk*, then *Almond Coating* mixture. For heavier coating, repeat.

9. Place coated onions in single layer on line dehydrator trays. Dehydrate on 110 degrees F for 6 - 8 hours, until *Almond Coating* is dry but onions are slightly moist.

10. Transfer to serving dish and serve immediately with your favorite sauce.

Spicy Cauliflower Chips

Prep Time: 5 minutes

Dehydrating Time: 12 - 24 hours

Servings: 2

INGREDIENTS

2 cups cauliflower florets (roughly chopped)

1 teaspoon raw oil (coconut, walnuts, almond, sesame, etc.)

1 tablespoon nutritional yeast

Celtic sea salt, to taste

Pinch cayenne pepper (optional)

INSTRUCTIONS

1. Cut larger cauliflower florets into smaller pieces. Add to medium mixing bowl or container with well-fitting lid.
2. Evenly sprinkle on oil, nutritional yeast, salt and cayenne pepper (optional).
3. Secure lid on bowl or container and shake well until cauliflower is evenly coated.
4. Line dehydrator trays with dehydrator or parchment sheets.
5. Add single layer of coated cauliflower to lined dehydrator sheet and place in dehydrator. Dehydrate on 115 degrees F for 12 - 24 hours, until desired crispiness is reached. Turn cauliflower over half way through ehydrating.
6. Remove from dehydrator and transfer to serving dish. Serve immediately.

Weight Loss Flax Crackers

Prep Time: 10 minutes

Dehydrating Time: 12 - 20 hours

Servings: 4

INGREDIENTS

2 cups ground flax seed

2/3 cup whole flax seed

1 1/3 cups raw sunflower seeds

1/2 cup raw black sesame seeds (or white sesame seeds)

Small bunch fresh parsley

1/4 teaspoon dried basil

1/4 teaspoon onion powder

1/4 teaspoon garlic powder

1 teaspoon Celtic sea salt

2 2/3 cups water

INSTRUCTIONS

1. Place parchment paper or dehydrator sheets on two dehydrator trays.
2. Finely mince fresh parsley. Add to large mixing bowl with seeds, salt and spices. Mix until well combined.
3. Spread batter on prepared sheets. Place trays in dehydrator and set to 120 degrees F for 1 hour. Reduce temperature to 105 degrees F for remainder of dehydrating time.

4. After 4 hours dehydrating time, remove trays from dehydrator and use knife to score crackers in preferred shape and size. Place back in dehydrator and continue dehydrating another 4 hours.
5. Remove trays from dehydrator. Peel crackers from sheets and break apart along score lines. Place crackers directly on dehydrator tray and continue dehydrating another 4 - 12 hours, depending on desired crispness.
6. Remove crackers from dehydrator and serve with your favorite raw dips, spreads and salsas. Or store in an airtight container up to 4 weeks.

Weight Zucchini Salsa

Prep Time: 10 minutes

Cook Time: 12 - 24 hours

Servings: 4

INGREDIENTS

1 medium tomato

1 medium onion

2 medium zucchini

1 cup ground flax seed

2 tablespoons coconut aminos (or raw apple cider vinegar)

1/2 teaspoon ground black pepper

1 teaspoon Celtic sea salt

INSTRUCTIONS

1. Place parchment paper or dehydrator sheets on two dehydrator trays.

2. Peel onion and chop. Chop zucchini and tomato. Add to food processor or high-speed blender with flax meal, coconut aminos or vinegar, salt and pepper. Process until well ground, about 2 minutes.

3. Spread batter on prepared sheets. Place trays in dehydrator and set to 120 degrees F for 1 hour. Reduce temperature to 105 degrees F for remainder of dehydrating time.

4. After 4 hours dehydrating time, remove trays from dehydrator and use knife to score crackers in preferred shape and size.

Place back in dehydrator and continue dehydrating another 4 hours.

5. Remove trays from dehydrator. Peel crackers from sheets and break apart along score lines. Place crackers directly on dehydrator tray and continue dehydrating another 4 - 12 hours, depending on desired crispness.

6. Remove crackers from dehydrator and serve with your favorite raw dips, spreads and salsas. Or store in an airtight container up to 4 weeks.

Quick Weight Loss Dates Spread

Prep Time: 5 minutes*

Servings: 4

INGREDIENTS

10 - 12 oz dried pitted dates

2 cups water

3 tablespoons raw cocoa powder

1/2 teaspoon ground cinnamon

1/4 teaspoon ground ginger

Ground black pepper, to taste

INSTRUCTIONS

1. *Soak dates in water overnight. Drain and reserve 1/4 cup liquid.

2. Add soaked dates, cocoa powder, cinnamon, ginger and black pepper to taste to food processor or high-speed blender. Pulse until chunky mixture forms. Add reserved liquid to reach desired consistency, if necessary.

3. Or add dates to medium mixing bowl with cocoa powder, cinnamon, ginger and black pepper to taste. Mash with large fork or potato masher for about 5 minutes, until chunky mixture forms. Add reserved liquid to reach desired consistency, if necessary.

4. Transfer to serving dish and serve with fruits, veggies, or raw crackers and breads.

All Chopped Creamy Dish

Prep Time: 15 minutes*

Servings: 2

INGREDIENTS

3 mature coconuts

1 1/2 cups water

6 clementines or tangerines (about 1 cup segments)

1 cup fresh pineapple (chopped)

1 cup pecans (chopped)

1 cup fresh cherries (pitted)

INSTRUCTIONS

1. Remove coconut flesh from shells. Add 1 coconut and water to food processor or high-speed blender. Process until well blended and fairly smooth, about 1 - 2 minutes.

2. Strain mixture through nut milk bag, cheesecloth or strainer into container. Add coconut milk back to blender with flesh of 2nd coconut. Process again until well blended and thick, about 1 - 2 minutes.

3. Strain mixture through nut milk bag, cheesecloth or strainer into container. Reserve pulp and set aside to dry and dehydrate, then use as coconut flour.

4. *For thicker coconut cream, set aside thickened milk in refrigerator about 20 minutes and allow fat to separate. Remove coconut cream from refrigerator and scoop out risen fat into medium mixing bowl.

5. Or add coconut cream milk to medium mixing bowl. Peel oranges or tangerines and remove segments. Peel pineapple and chop. Cut cherries in half and pit. Chop pecans. Add to coconut cream.

6. Add remaining coconut flesh to clean food processor with shredding attachment and process, or grate with grater. Add coconut to mixture. Stir to combine.

7. Cover mixture and place in refrigerator for 2 hours. Remove and transfer to serving dishes.

8. Serve chilled.

Weight Loss Sweet Toss

Prep Time: 20 minutes*

Servings: 2

INGREDIENTS

1 cup raw almonds

1 tablespoon raw cocoa powder

1 tablespoon raw honey

1/8 teaspoon ground cinnamon

1/8 teaspoon vanilla

INSTRUCTIONS

1. Add almonds and honey to small mixing bowl and toss to combine.
2. Add cocoa, cinnamon and vanilla and toss to evenly coat.
3. Transfer to serving dish and serve immediately.

Weight Loss Coconut Pudding

Prep Time: 20 minutes

Servings: 4

INGREDIENTS

3 fresh coconuts (or 2 cups unsweetened flaked or shredded coconut)

1 cup water

1/4 - 1/2 cup raw honey (or dried pitted dates)

1 teaspoon vanilla

Water

INSTRUCTIONS

1. *Soak 1 1/2 cups flaked coconut and dates in enough water to cover in refrigerator overnight. Then drain, if using.
2. Or remove fresh coconut flesh from shells.
3. Add flesh of 1 fresh coconut or 3/4 cup soaked coconut, and water to high-speed blender. Process until well blended and fairly smooth, about 1- 2 minutes.
4. Strain mixture through nut milk bag, cheesecloth or strainer into container. Add coconut milk back to blender with flesh of 1 fresh coconut or remaining soaked coconut. Process again until well blended and fairly smooth, about 1 minute.
5. Strain mixture through nut milk bag, cheesecloth or strainer into container. Reserve pulp and set aside to dry and dehydrate, then use as coconut flour.
6. Add coconut cream, soaked dates and vanilla to food processor or high-speed blender. Process until smooth, about 1 minute.

7. Or add coconut cream to medium mixing bowl with raw honey and vanilla.

8. Add remaining fresh coconut flesh to food processer with shredding attachment and process, or shred with grater.

9. Add shredded fresh coconut or flaked coconut to coconut cream mixture and whisk until well combined.

10. Pour into serving dishes and serve immediately. Or refrigerate for 20 minutes and serve chilled.

Cranberry & Broccoli Slaw

Prep Time: 15 minutes*

Servings: 4

INGREDIENTS

1/2 head red cabbage (2 cups shredded)

2 broccoli stalks (2 cups shredded)

1/4 cup dried cranberries

1/4 cup raw sliced or slivered almonds

2 tablespoons raw sunflower seeds

2 green onions (scallions)

1 carrot

1 lemon

1/2 orange

2 tablespoons raw honey

2 tablespoons raw sesame oil (or coconut, walnut, almond oil, etc.)

2 tablespoons apple cider vinegar

1/2 teaspoon ground ginger

1 teaspoon ground white pepper (or black pepper)

1 teaspoon Celtic sea salt

INSTRUCTIONS

1. Add broccoli and carrot to food processor with shredding attachment, or grate with grater. Slice green onions. Shred cabbage. Add to large mixing bowl.

2. Add cranberries, almonds, sunflower seeds, honey, oil, vinegar, ginger, salt, pepper and squeeze of lemon and orange. Mix until well combined.

3. *Transfer mixture and for 90 minutes. Serve chilled.

Spicy Onion & Fresh Mint Salsa

Prep Time: 5 minutes*

Servings: 4

INGREDIENTS

2 cups fresh strawberries

1/2 small white onion

1/4 red bell pepper

Medium bunch fresh mint

1/2 lime

1/2 orange

1/2 teaspoon ground black pepper

INSTRUCTIONS

1. Remove strawberry stems and leaves, then finely dice. Add to medium mixing bowl.

2. Peel onion and finely dice. Remove mint leave s from stem then chiffon, or thinly slice. Add to strawberries with pepper and squeeze of lime and orange. Mix until well combined.

3. Transfer mixture to serving dish and serve immediately with raw chips. Or refrigerate for 20 minutes and serve chilled.

Low Carb Cauliflower Fillers

Prep time:

Cook time:

INGREDIENTS

1 head of cauliflower

3 tbsp extra virgin olive oil

¼ tsp Celtic sea salt

INSTRUCTIONS

1. Preheat oven to 425 degrees.

2. Cut the head of cauliflower down to smaller florets, about an inch or so in length.

3. In a large bowl, combine cauliflower, extra virgin olive oil and Celtic sea salt and mix.

4. Place the cauliflower on a baking sheet and roast for 1 hour. Turn the pieces 4 times during baking at 15 minute intervals.

5. Remove from oven and let cool. Serve.

Broccoli Blasts

Prep time: 15 minutes

Cook time: 20 minutes

INGREDIENTS

1 large bunch of broccoli

2 tbsp extra virgin olive oil

1 tbsp garlic powder

¼ tsp Celtic sea salt

INSTRUCTIONS

1. Preheat oven to 450 degrees. Cut the broccoli into florets.

2. In a large bowl, mix broccoli florets, extra virgin olive oil, garlic powder and Celtic sea salt.

3. Spread the broccoli over a baking sheet and roast for 20 minutes until the edges are crispy.

4. Remove from oven and let cool. Serve.

Fresh Coriander with Melons

Prep time: over 5 hours combined

INGREDIENTS

1 Juan canary melon

2 tsp ground coriander

1 tbsp organic maple syrup

4 tsp fresh coriander

fresh coriander leaves

INSTRUCTIONS

1. Mince the fresh coriander. Chop the melon into small pieces. Combine the melon chunks, ground coriander, maple syrup and 3 tsp fresh minced coriander, and stir thoroughly. Place the mixture in the refrigerator for 1 hour.

2. Remove the mixture from the refrigerator and puree in a blender or food processor. Strain and remove the solids.

3. Add 1 tsp fresh minced coriander to the mixture and stir. Place the mixture in a serving pie dish and place in the freezer for 4 hours.

4. Remove from the freezer and spoon out each serving, garnishing with fresh coriander leaves.

Low Carb Celery Snack

Prep Time: 5 minutes

Cook Time: 5 minutes

Servings: 2

INGREDIENTS

3 celery stalks

2 tablespoons raisins

Cashew Butter

1 cup cashews

1 teaspoon coconut oil

1/2 teaspoon ground cinnamon

INSTRUCTIONS

1. Add cashews, cinnamon, and coconut oil to food processor or bullet blender. Process until smooth. Let mixture rest between periods of processing to reach desired consistency, if necessary.
2. Cut celery stakes into thirds and fill wells with *Cashew Butter*. Place raisins on cashew butter.
3. Serve room temperature. Or refrigerate 10 minutes and serve chilled.

Hot Chicken Paprika Wings

Prep Time: 5 minutes

Cook Time: 10 minutes

Servings: 4

INGREDIENTS

8 oz boneless skinless chicken

1/2 cup almond meal

1 teaspoon flax meal

1 teaspoon paprika

1/2 teaspoon cayenne pepper

1/2 teaspoon red pepper flakes

1/2 teaspoon ground black pepper

1/2 teaspoon sea salt

1 egg

1 jalapeño pepper

2 garlic cloves

2 oz organic spicy brown mustard

Coconut oil (for cooking)

INSTRUCTIONS

1. Heat a medium skillet over medium high heat. Lightly coat pan with coconut oil.

2. Slice chicken into 1x1 inch strips. Arrange slices between 2 sheets of parchment and pound with kitchen mallet or rolling pin to flatten slightly. Place flattened pieces between two paper towels to absorb excess moisture.

3. In a shallow dish, blend almond meal, flax meal, dry spices and salt.

4. Add egg , jalapeño and peeled garlic to food processor or bullet blender. Process until fairly smooth. Pour into shallow dish.

5. Dip chicken pieces into jalapeño egg, then dredge in seasoned almond meal.

6. Carefully place coated chicken pieces into hot oil and fry about 2 minutes, until golden brown and cooked through. Turn with tongs half way through.

7. Drain cooked chicken on paper towel, then transfer to serving dish.

8. Serve hot with spicy mustard.

Egg & Parsley Evening Glee

Prep Time: 10 minutes

Cook Time: 25 minutes

Servings: 6

INGREDIENTS

6 eggs

12 oz ground sausage (pork, chicken, etc.)

1 tablespoon dried parsley

2 teaspoons lemon zest

1/4 teaspoon ground nutmeg

1/4 teaspoon dried sage

Pinch sea salt

Pinch ground black pepper

1 egg

1/2 cup almond meal

Coconut oil (for cooking)

Mustard Sauce

1 egg yolk

1/4 cup coconut oil

1/4 cup organic mustard

2 tablespoons sweetener*

INSTRUCTIONS

1. Bring medium pot of lightly salted water to boil.
2. Carefully place eggs in pot with tongs. Boil eggs for about 10 minutes.
3. For *Mustard Sauce*, add yolk, coconut oil, mustard and sweetener to food processor and bullet blender. Process until emulsified, about 2 minutes. Transfer to serving dish and refrigerate about 15 minutes.
4. Heat small pot over medium heat. Add enough coconut oil to cover width of whole egg, about 2 1/2 inches.
5. Drain eggs and cool under cold running water. Once cool, peel off shells and set aside.
6. Add sausage to medium bowl with parsley, lemon zest, nutmeg, sage, salt and pepper. Mix to combine.
7. Wet hands and cover each whole, peeled egg with a layer of seasoned sausage. Work sausage around eggs and pat into even layer.
8. Pour almond meal into shallow dish. Whisk egg in small bowl. Roll sausage covered eggs in beaten egg, then dredge in almond meal.
9. Carefully place 2 eggs into hot oil and fry for 4 to 5 minutes, until browned and heated through. Turn half way through cooking with tongs.
10. Remove eggs with tongs or slotted spoon and place on paper towel to drain. Repeat with remaining eggs.
11. Serve hot with *Mustard Sauce*.

*stevia, raw honey or agave nectar

NOTE: For *Baked Scotch Eggs*, preheat oven to 400 degrees F and bake coated eggs on wire rack over sheet pan for about 15 minutes, until sausage is fully cooked.

Low Carb Spicy Egg & Coconut Salsa

Prep Time: 10 minutes

Cook Time: 15 minutes

Servings: 4

INGREDIENTS

3 egg whites

1 lb large shrimp

1 cup flaked coconut

1/2 teaspoon garlic powder

1/2 teaspoon ground white pepper (or ground black pepper)

1 teaspoon sea salt

Coconut oil (for cooking)

Mango Salsa

1 ripe mango

1/2 small white onion

1 small jalapeño

Juice of half lime

INSTRUCTIONS

1. Preheat oven to 425 degrees F. Line sheet pan with parchment paper. Or place oven-safe wire rack over sheet pan.
2. Add coconut to shallow dish.
3. Beat egg whites with salt, pepper and garlic powder in a large mixing bowl with hand mixer or whisk until light and fluffy.

4. Peel and devein shrimp. Leave tails on. Add shrimp to egg whites to coat.

5. Let excess egg white drain from shrimp, then add to coconut flakes. Toss to coat. Return shrimp to egg whites, then coconut flakes again. Press shrimp into coconut and coat well.

6. Place the shrimp on prepared sheet pan. Brush lightly with liquid coconut oil.

7. Place in oven and bake for 5 - 7 minutes. Then turn shrimp over, brush with coconut oil, and bake another 5 - 7 minutes, until coconut is golden brown and shrimp are bright pink.

8. For *Mango Salsa*, slice mango around pit. Peel and dice flesh. Peel and dice onion. Mince jalapeño, discarding seeds and stem. Add to small serving dish juice of half a lime. Mix to combine.

9. Remove shrimp from oven and allow to cool for a few minutes.

Serve warm with *Mango Salsa*

Spicy Green Devilled Eggs

Prep Time: 5 minutes

Cook Time: 10 minutes

Servings: 4

INGREDIENTS

8 eggs

1 avocado

1/2 teaspoon ground black pepper

1/2 teaspoon salt

2 oz natural ham

2 tablespoons fresh dill

INSTRUCTIONS

1. Bring medium pot of lightly salted water to boil. Gently add eggs to hot water with tongs and cook about 8 - 10 minutes.
2. Drain eggs in colander and cool in cold water.
3. Crack shells and peel eggs. Cut eggs in half lengthwise and scoop out yolks into small bowl. Arrange whites on platter with center hollows facing up.
4. Mash avocado, salt and pepper with egg yolks until smooth. Dice ham and dill, separately.
5. Scoop avocado blend into each egg white hollow and sprinkle with ham, then dill.
6. Refrigerate about 20 minutes. Serve chilled.

Hot Beef Quiche

Prep Time: 15 minutes

Cook Time: 25 minutes

Servings: 4

INGREDIENTS

Mini Burger Buns

1 1/2 cup raw cashews

1/3 cup coconut flour

1/4 cup almond flour

3 egg yolks

3 egg whites

1/4 cup coconut oil

1/4 cup nutmilk

1 teaspoon apple cider vinegar

1 teaspoon baking soda

1 teaspoon sea salt

Filling

8 oz ground meat (beef, chicken, turkey, etc.)

1 teaspoon ground black pepper

1 teaspoon paprika

1/2 teaspoon sea salt

1/2 small onion

1 mini dill pickle (or 1/2 large dill pickle)

Organic mustard

INSTRUCTIONS

1. Preheat oven to 325 degrees F. Line sheet pan with parchment paper or coat with coconut oil.

2. Preheat oven.

3. Place cashews, egg yolks, nut milk, coconut oil and vinegar in a food processor or bullet blender. Process until smooth. Add coconut flour, almond flour and salt. Process again until a smooth, wet dough forms.

4. Beat egg whites in medium bowl with hand mixer until stiff peaks form. Add wet dough to egg whites with and blend until combined.

5. Wet hands and shape dough into 12 mini buns, similar to burger patties. Wet hands in between each bun.

6. Place buns on prepared sheet pan **and bake for 10 -15 minutes, until golden and cooked through.**

7. **Heat large skillet or griddle over medium-high heat.**

8. **Mix ground meat with spices. Form into 12 mini patties. Place burgers on hot skillet or griddle and cook about 5 minutes, or until medium-well. Flip half way through cooking.**

9. **Remove buns from oven and allow to cool about 5 minutes.**

10. **Slices bun in half. Thinly slice onion and pickle. Place hamburger on bottom half of bun. Top with onion and pickle. Add mustard to taste. Top with top bun.**

11. **Serve warm.**

Desserts Recipes

Almond with Lemon Fillings

Prep Time: 15 minutes*

Servings: 8

INGREDIENTS

Crust

2 cups raw almonds

1/2 cup dried pitted dates

1/4 cup flaked or shredded coconut

Lemon Cheesecake Filling

3 cups raw cashews

3/4 cup fresh lemon juice (about 6 lemons)

3/4 cup raw honey (or 1 cup dried pitted dates)

3/4 cup raw coconut oil (or raw coconut or cacao butter, melted)

1 teaspoon vanilla

1/2 teaspoon Celtic sea salt

INSTRUCTIONS

1. *For *Crust*, soak almonds in enough water to cover overnight in refrigerator. Drain and rinse.

2. *For *Lemon Cheesecake Filling*, soak cashews in enough water to cover for 4 hours. Drain and rinse. Set aside. Soak dates in enough water to cover overnight in refrigerator, if using. Drain, reserving soaking liquid.

3. For *Crust*, place all ingredients in food processor or high-speed blender. Process until well ground and mixture sticks together, about 2 minutes.

4. Press *Crust* firmly into pie plate, cake pan or baking dish with hands. Set aside in refrigerator or freezer, if preferred.

5. For *Lemon Cheesecake Filling*, zest 1 lemon, then juice all lemons into clean food processor or high-speed blender. Add soaked cashews, vanilla, coconut oil or butter, salt, and honey or dates to clean food processor or high-speed blender. Process until smooth, about 2 - 3 minutes. Add enough date soaking liquid or water to reach desired consistency, if necessary. Mixture should be thick and smooth, but not runny.

6. Pour *Lemon Cheesecake Filling* into *Crust* and gently tap dish on counter to release any air bubbles. Smooth with spatula or back of a spoon, if needed.

7. *Cover pie with parchment, if preferred, and place in freezer at least 3 hours. Allow to warm slightly and serve chilled.

Nuts & Pecan Desserts

Prep Time: 15 minutes*

Servings: 8

INGREDIENTS

Crust

3/4 cup raw pecans

3/4 cup raw walnuts

1 1/4 cups dried pitted dates

1/4 cup flaked or shredded coconut

1/4 teaspoon Celtic sea salt

Pecan Filling

1 2/3 cups dried pitted dates

1/2 raw pecan pieces (or 3/4 raw pecan halves)

3/4 cup raw pecan halves (reserve)

1/4 cup raw coconut oil (or raw coconut or cacao butter, melted)

1 1/2 teaspoons vanilla

1 teaspoon ground cinnamon

1/4 teaspoon ground nutmeg

1/2 teaspoon Celtic sea salt

Water

INSTRUCTIONS

1. *For *Pecan Filling,* soak dates in enough water to cover for at least 4 hours, or overnight in refrigerator. Drain, reserving soaking liquid .

2. For *Crust*, place all ingredients in food processor or high-speed blender. Process until mixture is well ground and sticks together, about 2 - 3 minutes.

3. Press *Crust* firmly into pie plate, cake pan or baking dish with hands. Set aside in refrigerator or freezer, if preferred.

4. For *Pecan Filling*, add soaked dates to clean food processor or high-speed blender with pecan pieces, coconut oil or butter, vanilla, salt and spices. Process until thick smooth mixture forms, about 2 - 3 minutes. Add enough soaking liquid to reach desired consistency.

5. Pour *Pecan Filling* into *Crust* and smooth with spatula or back of a spoon. Top pie with reserve pecan halves.

6. Slice and serve immediately. Or refrigerate at least 1 hour and serve chilled.

Dried Dates Nuts Pie

Prep Time: 15 minutes*

Servings: 8

INGREDIENTS

Crust

1 cup raw almonds

1 cup raw pecans

1 cup raw walnuts

1 1/2 cups dried pitted dates

1/2 orange

1/2 teaspoon vanilla

1/2 teaspoon ground cinnamon

1/4 teaspoon ground nutmeg

1/4 teaspoon Celtic sea salt

Mincemeat Filling

2 cups dried pitted dates

1/2 cup raw almonds

1/2 cup dried apricots

1 1/2 oranges

1/2 lemon

2 tablespoons raw tahini

2 tablespoons raisins

2 tablespoons dried cherries (or goji or noni berries)

2 tablespoons raw pistachios

2 tablespoons shredded or flaked coconut

1 tablespoon chia seeds

1 teaspoon vanilla

1 teaspoon ground cinnamon

1/4 teaspoon ground nutmeg

1/4 teaspoon ground ginger

1/4 teaspoon Celtic sea salt

Water

INSTRUCTIONS

1. *For *Mincemeat Filling,* soak dates in enough water to cover for 1 hour, then drain.

2. For *Crust*, zest then juice orange into food processor or high-speed blender. Add all *Crust* ingredients and process until well ground and mixture sticks together, about 2 - 3 minutes.

3. Press *Crust* firmly into pie plate, cake pan or baking dish with hands. Set aside in refrigerator or freezer, if preferred.

4. For *Mincemeat Filling*, add chia to clean food processor or high-speed blender and process until finely ground, about 1 minute. Add raw almonds and process until finely ground, about 2 minutes.

5. Zest *then* juice oranges and lemon. Add to processor with soaked dates, tahini, salt and spices. Process until well ground and fairly smooth, about 2 minutes. Add apricots and pulse until roughly chopped.

6. Transfer to medium mixing bowl and stir in raisins and cherries. Mix to combine.

7. Pour *Mincemeat Filling* into *Crust* and smooth with spatula or back of a spoon. Roughly chop pistachios. Sprinkle chopped pistachios and coconut over pie.

8. Slice and serve immediately. Or refrigerate at least 1 hour and serve chilled.

Pecan with Pumpkin Feast

Prep Time: 15 minutes*

Servings: 8

INGREDIENTS

Crust

3/4 cup raw pecans

3/4 cup raw walnuts

1 1/4 cups dried pitted dates

Pinch Celtic sea salt

Pumpkin Filling

1 "pie pumpkin"

1 1/2 cups dried pitted dates

1/2 cup dried apricots

2 teaspoons ground cinnamon

1/2 teaspoon ground ginger

1/2 teaspoon vanilla

Water

INSTRUCTIONS

1. *For *Crust*, soak dates in enough water to cover for 1 hour, then drain.

2. *For *Pumpkin Filling,* soak dates in enough water to cover for at least 4 hours, or overnight in refrigerator. Drain, reserving soaking liquid .

3. For *Crust*, place all ingredients in food processor or high-speed blender. Process until mixture is well ground and sticks together, about 2 - 3 minutes.

4. Press *Crust* firmly into pie plate, cake pan or baking dish with hands. Set aside in refrigerator or freezer, if preferred.

5. For *Pumpkin Filling*, peel pumpkin and remove seeds and stringy innards. Chop pumpkin and add to clean food processor or high-speed blender with soaked dates, apricots, vanilla, cinnamon and ginger. Process until smooth, up to 5 minutes. Add enough soaking liquid to reach desired consistency. Mixture should be thick and smooth, but not runny.

6. Pour *Pumpkin Filling* into *Crust* and smooth with spatula or back of a spoon.

7. Slice and serve immediately. Or refrigerate at least 1 hour and serve chilled.

Nut Tart Berry Stuffs

Prep Time: 10 minutes*

Servings: 8

INGREDIENTS

1 1/2 cups fresh blueberries

Tart Shell

1 cup raw cashews (or raw walnuts)

1 cup raw macadamia nuts (or raw brazil nuts)

1/3 cup flaked or shredded coconut

1 cup dried pitted dates

1/2 teaspoon vanilla

Lemon Curd Filling

1 cup cashews

1/2 cup raw coconut butter (or raw cacao butter)

4 lemons

1/3 - 1/2 cup raw honey (or dried pitted dates)

Pinch Celtic sea salt

Pinch vanilla (optional)

Pinch ground turmeric (optional)

Water

INSTRUCTIONS

1. *For *Lemon Curd Filling*, soak cashews in enough water to cover at least 4 hours, or overnight in refrigerator. Drain and rinse. Set

aside. Soak dates in enough water to cover overnight in refrigerator, if using. Drain, reserving soaking liquid.

1. For *Tart Shell*, place all ingredients in food processor or high-speed blender. Process until well ground and mixture sticks together, about 2 minutes.

2. Press *Crust* firmly into tart pan or pie plate with hands. Set aside in refrigerator or freezer, if preferred.

3. For *Lemon Curd Filling*, zest 1 lemon, then juice all lemons into clean food processor or high-speed blender. Add soaked cashews, soaked dates or honey, salt, and vanilla and turmeric (optional). Process until smooth, about 2 minutes. Add enough soaking liquid or water to reach desired consistency. Mixture should be smooth, but not too runny.

4. Pour *Lemon Curd Filling* into *Crust* and smooth with spatula or back of a spoon. Tp pie with fresh blueberries.

5. Refrigerate at least 1 hour, until set. Slice and serve chilled

High Protein Crust

Prep Time: 25 minutes*

Servings: 8

INGREDIENTS

Topping

1/2 cup raw pecans

1/2 cup raw walnuts

1/2 cup raw almonds

Crust

1 cup raw almonds

1 cup raw pecans

1 cup raw walnuts

1 1/2 cups dried pitted dates

1 teaspoon vanilla

1/2 teaspoon ground cinnamon

1/2 teaspoon Celtic sea salt

Apple Filling

3 apples

1/4 - 1/3 cup dried pitted dates

1/2 lemon

2 tablespoons flax seeds

1 teaspoon vanilla

1 teaspoon ground cinnamon

1/2 teaspoon Celtic sea salt

Water

INSTRUCTIONS

1. *For *Apple Filling*, soak dates in enough water to cover for 1 hour, then drain.
2. For *Topping*, add nuts to food processor or high-speed blender. Pulse until finely chopped. Set aside.
3. For *Crust*, place all ingredients in food processor or high-speed blender. Process until well ground and mixture sticks together, about 2 - 3 minutes.
4. Press *Crust* firmly into pie plate, cake pan or baking dish with hands. Set aside in refrigerator or freezer, if preferred.
5. For *Apple Filling*, add flax to clean food processor or high-speed blender and process until finely ground, about 1 minute.
6. Peel and core apples, then roughly chop. Juice lemon and add to processor with 1/3 of apples, soaked dates, vanilla and salt. Process until smooth, about 2 minutes.
7. Add 1/2 of remaining apples and process until finely chopped, but still chunky. Add remaining apples and pulse until roughly chopped. Set aside 15 minutes.
8. Pour *Apple Filling* into *Crust* and smooth with spatula or back of a spoon. Evenly sprinkle *Topping* over pie to create top crust.
9. Slice and serve immediately. Or refrigerate at least 1 hour and serve chilled.

Sugar Free Crust with Peach Stuffing

Prep Time: 10 minutes*

Servings: 8

INGREDIENTS

Crust

1 cup raw pecans

1 cup raw walnuts

1 cup dried pitted dates

1/2 teaspoon vanilla

1/2 teaspoon ground cinnamon

1/4 teaspoon Celtic sea salt

Peach Filling

4 ripe peaches (or nectarines)

1 teaspoon ground cinnamon

1/2 teaspoon ground nutmeg

1/4 teaspoon vanilla

1/4 teaspoon ground ginger (optional)

INSTRUCTIONS

1. For *Crust*, place all ingredients in food processor or high-speed blender. Process until well ground and mixture sticks together, about 2 minutes.

2. Press *Crust* firmly into pie plate, cake pan or baking dish with hands. Set aside in refrigerator or freezer, if preferred.

3. For *Peach Filling*, cut peaches in half and remove pit. Thinly slice and add to large mixing bowl. Sprinkle on spices and salt. Gently toss to coat evenly.

4. Pour *Peach Filling* and press into *Crust*.

5. Slice and serve immediately. Or refrigerate at least 1 hour and serve chilled.

Macadamia with Berry Filling

Prep Time: 15 minutes*

Servings: 8

INGREDIENTS

Crust

1 1/2 cups raw hazelnuts (or macadamia nuts)

1 cup raw almonds

1/4 cup dried pitted dates

1 teaspoon ground cinnamon

Blueberry Filling

4 cups pitted cherries (fresh or thawed)

1/4 cup raw coconut oil (or raw coconut or cacao butter, melted)

1/4 dried pitted dates

1/2 teaspoon vanilla

Pinch Celtic sea salt

INSTRUCTIONS

1. *For *Crust*, soak dates in enough water to cover for 1 hour, then drain.
2. Add nuts to food processor or high-speed blender and process until coarsely ground, about 1 minute. Add dates and cinnamon and process until mixture is well ground and sticks together, about 1 minute.
3. Press *Crust* firmly into pie plate, cake pan or baking dish with hands. Set aside in refrigerator or freezer, if preferred.

4. *For *Cherry Filling*, pit whole cherries, if using.

5. Add 1/3 of pitted cherries to clean food processor or high-speed blender with coconut oil or butter, dates, vanilla and salt. Process until smooth, about 1 - 2 minutes.

6. Add 1/2 of remaining cherries to processor and pulse to roughly chop.

7. Pour *Cherry Filling* into *Crust* and smooth with spatula or back of a spoon. Roughly chop or halve remaining cherries. Sprinkle remaining cherries over pie.

8. *Refrigerate at least 1 hour, until set. Slice and serve chilled. Or allow to warm slightly and serve.

Creamy Blueberry Filling

Prep Time: 15 minutes*

Servings: 8

INGREDIENTS

Crust

1 cup raw almonds (or raw pecans)

1 cup dried pitted dates

1 1/2 cups flaked or shredded coconut

1/2 lemon

1 teaspoon vanilla

Pinch Celtic sea salt

Blueberry Filling

2 cups blueberries (fresh or thawed)

1/2 cup raw coconut oil (or raw coconut or cacao butter, melted)

1/4 cup cashew butter(or 1/2 cup raw cashews)

1/4 - 1/3 cup dried pitted dates

1/2 lemon

1 teaspoon vanilla

1/4 teaspoon Celtic sea salt

INSTRUCTIONS

1. For *Crust*, add almonds to food processor or high-speed blender and process until finely ground, about 2 minutes. Zest *then* juice lemon in to processer with remaining *Crust* ingredients. Process until mixture is well ground and sticks together, about 2 minutes.

2. Press *Crust* firmly into pie plate, cake pan or baking dish with hands. Set aside in refrigerator or freezer, if preferred.

3. For *Blueberry Filling*, zest *then* juice lemon into clean food processor or high-speed blender. Add raw cashews and blend until smooth, if using.

4. Or add cashew butter, dates, and coconut oil or butter to processor. Process until smooth, about 1 - 2 minutes.

5. Add 1 1/2 cups blueberries, vanilla and salt to processor. Process until thick smooth mixture forms, about 1 minute.

6. Pour *Blueberry Filling* into *Crust* and smooth with spatula or back of a spoon. Sprinkle remaining blueberries over pie.

7. Slice and serve immediately. Or refrigerate at least 1 hour and serve chilled.

Sugar Free Carrot Bakes

Prep Time: 10 minutes*

Servings: 8

INGREDIENTS

Carrot Cake

2 - 3 large carrots

2 cups raw walnuts

1/2 cup raisins (or dried apricots)

1/2 cup flaked or shredded coconut

2 tablespoons raw pumpkin seeds

1/4 cup raw honey (or dried pitted dates)

1 teaspoon vanilla

1 teaspoon ground cinnamon

1/4teaspoon ground nutmeg

1/4 teaspoon ground ginger (optional)

Cashew Cream Icing

1 cup raw cashews

1/2 large lemon

2 tablespoons raw honey (or dried pitted dates)

1 teaspoon vanilla

Water

INSTRUCTIONS

1. *For *Cashew Cream Icing*, separately soak cashews and dates (if using) in enough water to cover for 2 hours. Drain dates. Drain and rinse cashews.

2. For *Carrot Cake*, add carrots to food processor or high-speed blender and pulse to roughly chop. Add all *Carrot Cake* ingredients and process until coarsely ground but still slightly chunky, about 1 minute.

3. Transfer mixture to cake or baking pan and press firmly with hands.

4. For *Cashew Cream Icing*, juice lemon and add to clean food processor or high-speed blender with soaked cashews, soaked dates or honey, and vanilla. Process until smooth, about 2 minutes. Add enough date soaking liquid or water to reach desired consistency.

5. Spread *Cashew Cream Icing* over *Carrot Cake* and place in refrigerator at least 2 hours.

6. Slice and serve chilled. Or allow to warm slightly and serve.

Dried Chocolate Brown Cake

Prep Time: 10 minutes*

Servings: 8

INGREDIENTS

Chocolate Cake

1 1/2 cups raw pecans

1 1/2 cups raw walnuts

1 1/2 cups dried pitted dates

1 1/2 cups raisins (or dried apricots or other dried fruit)

1/3 cup raw cocoa powder

2 teaspoons vanilla

Chocolate Icing

1 cup raw cashews

4 tablespoons raw honey (or dried pitted dates)

2 tablespoons raw cocoa powder

1/2 teaspoon vanilla

Water

INSTRUCTIONS

1. *For *Chocolate Icing*, separately soak cashews and dates (if using) in enough water to cover for 2 hours. Drain dates. Drain and rinse cashews.

2. For *Chocolate Cake*, add pecans and walnuts to food processor or high-speed blender. Process until coarsely ground, about 1 minute.

3. Add dates and process until finely ground, about 1 minute. Repeat with raisins, then cocoa and vanilla.

4. Process all ingredients until dough comes together. Transfer mixture to cake or baking pan and press firmly with hands.

5. For *Chocolate Icing*, add soaked cashews, soaked dates or honey, cocoa and vanilla to clean food processor or high-speed blender. Process until smooth, about 2 minutes. Add enough date soaking liquid or water to reach desired consistency.

6. Pour *Chocolate Icing* over *Chocolate Cake* and smooth with spatula or back of a spoon.

7. Refrigerate at least 1 hour, until cake is firm. Slice and serve chilled. Or allow to warm slightly and serve.

Rich Fruit Flax Dessert

Prep Time: 10 minutes*

Dehydrating Time: 14 - 16 hours

Servings: 8

INGREDIENTS

Banana Bread

1 cup raw almonds

2 ripe bananas

2 sweet apples

2 carrots

1/2 cup flax meal (or flax seeds)

1/4 cup dried pitted dates

1/4 cup chopped walnuts

INSTRUCTIONS

1. Add whole flax to food processor or high-speed blender, if using. Process until finely ground, about 2 minutes.

2. Transfer flax meal to medium mixing bowl.

3. Add almonds to processor and process until finely ground, about 2 minutes. Add to flax.

4. Peel and core apples. Peel bananas. Roughly chop and add to processor. Process until puréed, about 2 minutes. Add to almond and flax meal.

5. Add carrots and dates to processor. Process until puréed, about 2 - 3 minutes. Add enough water to reached desired consistency, if necessary.

6. Add carrot and date purée to mixing bowl with walnuts. Mix to combine. Mixture should stick together. Add flax meal and/or water to reach desired consistency, if necessary.

7. Line dehydrator tray with dehydrator or parchment sheet.

8. Form mixture into loaves and place on lined dehydrator tray. Dehydrate at 118 degrees F for 14 - 16 hours. Until the outside is firm to the touch but the inside is still moist.

9. Remove from dehydrator and slice. Transfer to serving dish serve immediately. Or store in airtight container.

Creamy Vanilla Scoop

Prep Time: 15 minutes

Dehydrating Time: 24 hours

Servings: 12

INGREDIENTS

2 1/2 cups flaked or shredded coconut

1/3 cup dried pitted dates

1/3 cup water

1/2 teaspoon vanilla

Pinch Celtic sea salt

INSTRUCTIONS

1. Add 1 1/4 cups coconut to food processor or high-speed blender. Process until smooth and creamy, up to 5 minutes. Scrape down sides of bowl as necessary.

2. Add dates, water, vanilla and salt to processor. Process until smooth, about 2 minutes.

3. Transfer mixture to medium mixing bowl. Add remaining coconut and mix until well combined.

4. Line dehydrator tray with dehydrator or parchment sheets.

5. Use scoop or tablespoon to drop cookies onto lined dehydrator trays. Dehydrate at 118 degrees F for about 24 hours. Until the outside is dry to the touch but the inside is still moist.

6. Remove from dehydrator and transfer to serving dish. Serve immediately. Or store in airtight container.

Energy Reviving Almond Slices

Prep Time: 10 minutes*

Dehydrating Time: 12 - 24 hours

Servings: 12

INGREDIENTS

1 1/2 cups raw almond flour

2 cups raw almonds

1 cup flaked or shredded coconut

1/2 cup raw honey (or dried pitted dates)

1/2 cup dried apricots or golden raisins (optional)

1 teaspoon vanilla

1/4 teaspoon Celtic sea salt

Water

INSTRUCTIONS

1. *Soak dates in enough water to cover overnight in refrigerator, if using. Drain, reserving soaking liquid.
2. Add 1 1/2 cups almonds to food processor or high-speed blender. Process until finely ground, about 2 minutes.
3. Add coconut to processor and process until finely ground, about 1 minute.
4. Add soaked dates or honey, vanilla, salt, and apricots or raisins (optional) to processor. Process until well ground, about 1 - 2 minutes. Transfer mixture to mixing bowl.

5. Add almond flour and remaining 1/2 cup raw almonds. Mix well to combine. Add date soaking liquid to reach desired consistency. Dough should be moist and stick together.

6. Line dehydrator trays with dehydrator or parchment sheets.

7. Form mixture into loaves and place on dehydrator or parchment sheets.

8. Place in dehydrator and dehydrate at 118 degrees F for about 8 hours.

9. Remove from dehydrator and cut into 3/4 inch slices. Turn slices on sides and place directly on dehydrator tray. Continue dehydrating 4 - 16 hours, depending on desired crispiness.

10. Remove from dehydrator and transfer to serving dish. Serve immediately. Or store in airtight container.

Sugar Free Gingerly Pudding

Prep Time: 20 minutes*

Servings: 2

INGREDIENTS

1 young coconut (about 1 cup coconut meat and 1 cup coconut water)

2 - 4 tablespoons raw honey (or pitted dates)

1 1/2 inch piece fresh ginger

1/2 teaspoon ground ginger

1 teaspoon vanilla

Water (optional)

INSTRUCTIONS

1. Soak dates in enough water to cover for at least 4 hours, or overnight in refrigerator (if using). Drain.
2. Remove flesh from fresh coconut and add to high-speed blender with 1 cup coconut water. Process until well blended and fairly smooth, about 1 - 2 minutes.
3. Peel ginger and grate into processor. Add vanilla, ground ginger, and honey or dates. Process until smooth, about 1 minute.
4. Transfer to serving dish and serve immediately or refrigerate at least 20 minutes and serve chilled.

Almond Vanilla Banana Pudding

Prep Time: 10 minutes

Cook Time: 30 minutes

Servings: 12

INGREDIENTS

Banana Bread

1 cup of almond flour

2 eggs

2 overripe bananas

1/4 cup sweetener*

2 tablespoons coconut oil

1 tablespoon baking powder

1 tablespoon cinnamon

1 teaspoon nutmeg

1 teaspoon vanilla

1/2 teaspoon of sea salt

Banana Custard

13 oz (1 can) full-fat coconut milk

6 egg yolks

1 overripe banana

1/4 cup sweetener*

1/4 cup raisins

1/2 cup dried pitted dates

2 tablespoons tapioca starch/flour

2 teaspoons vanilla

1 teaspoon cinnamon

Pinch sea salt

INSTRUCTIONS

1. Preheat oven to 350 degrees F. Line muffin pan with paper liners or coat with coconut oil.
2. In medium mixing bowl, beat 2 eggs, 2 bananas, 2 tablespoons oil and 1/4 cup sweetener with hand mixer or whisk.
3. In separate mixing bowl, add 1 cup almond flour, 1 tablespoon baking powder,1 tablespoon cinnamon, 1 teaspoon nutmeg, 1 teaspoon vanilla and 1/2 teaspoon salt.
4. Pour banana mixture into flour mixture and mix well.
5. Pour batter into muffin pan and bake for about 15 minutes, or until golden brown, risen and firm.
6. While muffins cook, add coconut milk, egg yolks, banana, sweetener, vanilla, cinnamon and salt to medium bowl and blend briefly with hand mixer or whisk.
7. Pour into medium pot and heat over medium heat. Chop dates and add to pot with raisins.
8. Stir in tapioca flour. Stir as *Banana Custard* thickens, about 5 minutes. Remove from heat.
9. Remove muffins from oven and turn out onto cutting board.
10. Increase oven to 375 degrees F. Lightly coat square or rectangular baking dish with coconut oil.
11. Carefully remove paper liners and roughly chop muffins. Add muffin chunks to baking dish. Pour banana custard over chopped muffins.
12. Place dish in oven and bake for 15 minutes.

13. Remove and allow to cool for 15 minutes before serving.

14. Serve warm or room temperature.

*stevia, raw honey or agave nectar

Creamy Almond & Coconut Pie

Prep Time: 20 minutes*

Cook Time: 20 minutes

Servings: 8

INGREDIENTS

Crust

1/2 cup soft nuts**

1 cup almond flour

2 teaspoons sweetener***

1/4 - 1/2 cupcoconut oil

Filling

26oz (2 cans) full-fat coconut milk

2 eggs

1/2 cup arrowroot powder

1/4 cup sweetener*

1 tablespoon vanilla

1 cup flaked coconut

Pinch sea salt

INSTRUCTIONS

1. Preheat oven to 350 degrees F. Lightly coast pie plate with coconut oil.

2. Grind nutsinto coarse meal with food processor or bullet blender. Add to small bowl with almond flour, 2 tablespoons

sweetener and enough coconut oil to bring together soft but crumbly dough.

3. Press dough into pie plate and bake about 10 - 15 minutes, until crust becomes golden.

4. Remove crust from oven and allow to cool. Turn off oven.

5. Add coconut milk, eggs, arrowroot powder, sweetener,vanilla and salt to medium pot. Heat pot over medium heat and bring to a boil. Stir constantly as mixture thickens.

6. Stir in 1/2 cupshredded coconut. Then pour the filling over the crust.

7. *Refrigerate pie until filling is set, about 4 hours.

8. Heat medium pan over medium heat. Add 1/2 cup flaked coconut and toast about 5 minutes. Stir frequently to prevent burning.

9. Sprinkle toasted coconut over pie and serve chilled.

NOTE: Line springform pan with parchment and bake crust, then fill with coconut cream filling for another version of **Coconut Cream Pie**.

*coconut flakes, pecans, walnuts, cashews or brazil nuts
**stevia, raw honey or agave nectar

New Yorkshire Pecan Chess Pies

Prep Time: 20 minutes

Cook Time: 25 minutes

Servings: 6

INGREDIENTS

Crust

1 1/2 cups almond flour

1/2 cup pecans

1 egg

2 tablespoons coconut oil

1/4 teaspoon sea salt

Filling

1 cup full-fat coconut milk

2 cups pecans

1 cup dried pitted dates

1/2 cup sweetener*

2 eggs

2 egg yolks

1 1/2 tablespoons arrowroot powder

2 tablespoons coconut oil

1 teaspoon vanilla

INSTRUCTIONS

1. Preheat oven to 350 degrees F. Coat 6 mini pie plates or pie pans with coconut oil. Bring small pot of water to boil, leaving room for dates.

2. Add dates to boiling water for about 5 - 10 minutes, until tender. Then drain.

3. For *Crust*, process pecans in food processor or bullet lender until well ground. Add to small mixing bowl with almond flour and salt. Mix in oil and egg until dough forms.

4. Press dough into pie plates with hand or wooden spoon. Bake about 10 minutes, until golden. Remove pie shells from oven and set aside.

5. Chop 1 cup pecans and set aside

6. For *Filling*, process softened dates in food processor or bullet blender with about half of coconut milk. Add to medium mixing bowl with remainingcoconut milk, sweetener, eggs, egg yolks, coconut oil, vanilla and arrowroot powder. Beat with hand mixer or whisk until combined and a bit airy. Mix in chopped pecans.

7. Pour batter into mini pie crusts. Top with whole pecans and bake for 20 - 25 minutes, until filling is set.

8. Remove pies and let cool about 20 minutes before serving.

9. Serve warm. Or refrigerate and serve cold. Also great at room temperature.

stevia, raw honey or agave nectar

NOTE: For large **Pecan ChessPie**, bake in 9-inch pie plate for 45 - 55 minutes, or until center is set.

Low Carb Almond & Cashew Balls

Prep Time: 10 minutes

Cook Time: 10 minutes

Servings: 12

INGREDIENTS

1/2 cup almond butter

1/2 cup almonds

1/4 cup cashews

1 tablespoon cocoa powder

1 tablespoon ground chia seed (or flax meal)

5 dried pitted dates

3/4 cup flaked coconut

2 tablespoons sweetener*

1 teaspoon cinnamon

INSTRUCTIONS

1. Heat small pot over high heat. Add cashews and enough water to cover. Boil cashews until softened, about 8 minutes.

2. Add softened cashews to food processor or bullet blender with sweetener, and process until smooth. Add water to thin if mixture is too thick or chunky. Scrape into small mixing bowl.

3. Chop dates and almonds by hand or in food processor or bullet blender. Add to cashew cream with almond butter and mix together.

4. Add cocoa powder, chia or flax meal, coconut and cinnamon, and blend.

5. Add 1 tablespoon at a time of almond butter or cocoa powder to get mixture to perfect consistency to hold together as a ball.
6. Use mini scoop or tablespoon to portion twelve servings. Roll each serving into a ball. Place balls onparchment covered half sheet pan or plate and refrigerate for about 20 minutes.
7. Serve chilled or room temperature.

*stevia, raw honey or agave nectar

Baked Cranberries

Prep Time: 5 minutes

Cook Time: 25 minutes

Servings: 4

INGREDIENTS

2 ripe peaches

1/4 cup walnuts

1/4 cup dried cranberries

2 tablespoons sweetener*

Juice of 1 orange

Zest of 1 orange

1 teaspoon cinnamon

1/2 teaspoon nutmeg

1/2 teaspoon ground allspice

INSTRUCTIONS

1. Preheat oven to 375degrees F.
2. Slice peaches in half and remove pit. Place peach halves into glass or ceramic baking dish just big enough for them to fit snuggly.
3. Chop walnuts and toss with cranberries, sweetener, spices, juice and zest of orange in small bowl.
4. Fill peach halves with fruit and nut mixture. Pour excess liquid over peaches.
5. Bake in oven for about 20 - 25 minutes, until peaches are soften and lightly browned.

6. Remove from oven and let cool about 5 minutes.

7. Serve warm or room temperature.

stevia, raw honey or agave nectar

Vanilla Coconut with Cashew Mascarpone

Prep Time: 20 minutes*

Cook Time: 10 minutes

Servings: 8

INGREDIENTS

Lady Fingers

1/3 cup coconut flour

3 tablespoons arrowroot powder

4 eggs

1/4 cup sweetener**

1/2 teaspoon baking powder

1/2 teaspoon vanilla

2 tablespoons instant espresso (or instant coffee)

3/4 cup water

2 tablespoons cocoa powder

Cashew Mascarpone

2 cups cashews

2 tablespoons sweetener**

1 teaspoon lemon juice

1 teaspoon vanilla

Water

INSTRUCTIONS

1. *Soak 2 cups cashews in water overnight. Drain and rinse.

2. Preheat oven to 400 degrees F. Line two sheet pans with parchment paper. Fit pastry bag with 1/2 inch round tube, or cut 1/4 inch corner off sturdy kitchen storage bag (like Ziploc®).

3. Beat egg yolks, 1/4 cup sweetener and 1/2 teaspoon vanilla until thick and pale.

4. In separate bowl beat egg whites to stiff peaks with hand mixer or whisk in medium bowl. Fold half of egg whites into egg yolk mixture. Then sift in coconut flour, arrowroot powder and baking powder. Fold in remaining egg whites.

5. Scoop batter into pastry bag or storage bag. Place in tall wide contain and fold open end of bag over edge of container for greater ease.

6. Pipe 5 inch lady fingers onto parchment lined sheet pans about 2 inches apart. Bake for 8 minutes.

7. Remove cookies from oven and transfer full parchment sheet onto wire rack to cool completely. Do not try to remove warm cookies from parchment.

8. Process soaked cashews in food processor or bullet blender with sweetener, lemon juice, vanilla, and just enough water to smooth.

9. Bring 3/4 cup water just under a boil. Dissolve instant espresso or coffee in water and add to shallow dish.

10. Remove cooled lady fingers form parchment. Dip and roll each cookie in espresso, then arrange in single layer in glass baking dish. Cut cookies to fit into tight layer.

11. Dollop and spread on half of *Cashew Mascarpone*. Then add another layer of espresso dipped lady fingers. Top with last half of *Cashew Mascarpone* and sift on cocoa powder.

12. *Refrigerate at least 30 - 60 minutes.

13. Slice and serve chilled.

*stevia, raw honey or agave nectar

Very Berry Mixed Trifle

Prep Time: 10 minutes

Cook Time: 25 minutes

Servings: 12

INGREDIENTS

Cake

1 cup almond flour

1 cup coconut flour

3/4 cup coconut milk

4 eggs

1/2 cup sweetener*

1/2 cup coconut oil

2 tablespoons vanilla

2 teaspoons baking soda

Filling

1 cup coconut cream

2 tablespoons sweetener*

1 cup strawberries

1/2 cup blueberries

1/2 cup raspberries

1/2 cup blackberries

Juice of orange half

Juice of lemon half

Zest of orange half

Zest of lemon half

1/4 cup pistachios

INSTRUCTIONS

1. Preheat oven to 350 degrees F. Line muffin pan with paperliner or coat with coconut oil.
2. In large mixing bowl, beat eggs and coconut milk until light and airy. Beat in sweetener, oil and vanilla.
3. Sift in almond flour, coconut flour and baking soda. Mix until well combined.
4. Use ice cream scoop or spoon to scoop batter into muffin pan. Fill each cup 1/2 - 2/3 full with batter.
5. Bake in for about 15 minutes, until firm but springy in the center.
6. Remove cupcakes from oven and turn out onto wire rack or plate. Allow to cool for about 10 minutes and remove paper liners.
7. Dice strawberries and add to medium bowl with blueberries, raspberries, blackberries, lemon and orange zests and juices. Toss to combine.
8. In small bowl, mixi coconut cream with 2 tablespoon sweetener.
9. Slice cupcake in half to create top and bottom. Dollop coconut cream onto bottom half, then top with a spoonful of fruit. Drain juice from spoon before adding to cake.
10. Place cupcake top on top of fruit. Press down slightly. Add another dollop of coconut cream and another spoonful of fruit. Repeat with remaining cupcakes.
11. Serve room temperature. Or chill for 30 minutes and serve.

NOTE: Bake cake in 3 round cake pans for20 minutes, then layer with cream and berries and stack for **Mixed Berry Trifle Cake**.

*stevia, raw honey or agave nectar

Vanilla Cocoa Almond Biscotti

Prep Time: 15 minutes

Cook Time: 35* minutes

Servings: 6

INGREDIENTS

1 cup almond flour

1/2 cup coconut flour

1/2 cup sweetener*

1/3 cup almonds

2 tablespoons cocoa powder

1 teaspoon vanilla

1/2 teaspoon baking soda

1/4 teaspoon sea salt

INSTRUCTIONS

1. Preheat oven to 350 degrees F. Line sheet pan with parchment paper. Heat medium pan over medium heat.
2. Add almonds to hot dry pan and toast for about 5 minutes, until aromatic. Stir frequently. Remove from heat and set aside.
3. In medium mixing bowl, blend almond flour, coconut flour, cocoa powder, baking soda and saltwith hand mixer or whisk.
4. Beat in sweetener and vanilla until well combined and thick, sticky dough forms. Mix in toasted almonds with wooden spoon.
5. Formdough into flattened, uniform moundabout 1 inch thick on sheet pan. Pat down mound to keep any almonds from sticking out.

6. Bake for about 15 minutes . Remove and allow to cool for about 15 minutes.

7. Use a very sharp serrated knife to carefully cut biscotti log into 1/2 - 2/3 inch slices. Hold onto the mound and cut on a diagonal. If it becomes crumbly, stick it back together.

8. Lace slice on sides and return to oven for 15 minutes.

9. Try to cut so that you're holding on to the edges of the log to keep it from crumbling. If parts come apart, you can stick them back together as the mixture is still kind of sticky.

10. Lay the biscotti flat and return to oven for 15 minutes.

11. *Turn oven off and leave oven door open a crack. Allow the biscotti to cool and dry for at least 2 hours.

12. Serve room temperature.

raw honey, agave nectar, maple syrup, or any combination

Low Carb Wheat-Free Chocó Cake

Prep Time: 15 minutes

Cook Time: 30 minutes

Servings: 8

INGREDIENTS

16 oz organic bittersweet chocolate

1/4 cup cocoa powder

6 eggs

1 cup coconut oil

3/4 cup sweetener*

2 tablespoons water

2 teaspoons vanilla

1/4 teaspoon sea salt

INSTRUCTIONS

1. Preheat oven to 275 degrees F. Coat 2 mini spring form pans with coconut oil, then dust with cocoa powder, and cover the outside base of the pans with aluminum foil. Or line muffin pan with paper liners, or leave bare and coat liners or bare pan with coconut oil and dust with cocoa powder.

2. Slowly melt chocolate and coconut oil over a double boiler, heated over medium heat. Do not boil water in bottom of double boiler. Stir frequently.

3. Remove from heat once chocolate is melted and beat in sweetener, water, vanilla, salt and any remaining cocoa powder with hand mixer or whisk.

4. Beat in eggs one at a time until thoroughly incorporated.
5. Pour batter into vessels and bake for about 25 - 30 minutes, until set. Cakes will still appear a bit glossy and wet in the middle.
6. Cool for 30 minutes, then refrigerate at least 2 hours before serving.
7. Cut springform cakes with a knife warmed until hot running water, then dried.
8. Serve chilled or room temperature.

maple syrup, raw honey or agave nectar

Spicy Pumpkin Puree Cakes

Prep Time: 5 minutes

Cook Time: 15 minutes

Servings: 12

INGREDIENTS

3/4 cup coconut flour

4 eggs

1/4 cup coconut oil

1/2 cup sweetener*

1/2 cup pumpkin purée

1 teaspoon baking soda

1 tablespoon ground cinnamon

1 tablespoon ground ginger

1 tablespoon ground nutmeg

1 tablespoon ground black pepper

1 teaspoon vanilla

1/2 teaspoon sea salt

1/4 cup pumpkin seeds

INSTRUCTIONS

1. Preheat oven to 350 degrees F. Lightly coat 4 mini cake pans or mini loaf pans with coconut oil, or line with parchment paper.

2. Sift coconut flour, baking soda, salt and spices into large mixing bowl.

3. In medium mixing bowl, beat egg whites to soft peaks with hand mixer or whisk. About 5 minutes.

4. Then beat in yolks, oil, sweetener and pumpkin purée. Mix wet ingredients into dry blend until combined.

5. Pour batter into mini cake loaf pans and sprinkle on pumpkin seeds.

6. Bake for 20 - 25 minutes, or until firm but springy in the center and browned. A toothpick inserted into the middle should come out clean.

7. Remove from oven and allow to cool for 5 minutes before serving.

8. Serve warm or room temperature.

NOTE: For large **Pumpkin Spice Cake**, oil large loaf pan or springform pan and bake 40 - 45 minutes.

* raw honey, agave nectar or maple syrup

www.ingramcontent.com/pod-product-compliance
Lightning Source LLC
Chambersburg PA
CBHW070103290526
45789CB00005B/1904